The New Normal

The New Normal

a widow's guide to grief

Dr. Olga Lavalle

Copyright © 2018 by Dr. Olga Lavalle

All rights reserved. No part of this publication may be reproduced, distributed or transmitted in any form or by any means, without prior written permission.

Dr Olga Lavalle

Wollongong, New South Wales, Australia 2500

Ph: +61 0416261765

www.olgalavalle.com

Publisher's Note: This is a work of personal research. Locales and public names are sometimes used for atmospheric purposes. Any resemblance to actual people, living or dead, or to businesses, companies, events, institutions, or locales is completely coincidental.

Dr. Olga Lavalle. – 1st ed. ISBN 978-0-9874683-9-0

As a clinical psychologist Dr. Olga Lavalle is educated and well versed in hearing people's tales of grief. It's fair to say she is well equipped to listen, and offer practical tools to help manage the heartache.

But when her own heart was broken with one phone call, she had no idea how she was supposed to react in that moment…

This heartfelt book is a step by step guide. You'll discover a kindred spirit in Dr. Olga, she understands what you're going through. Help manage the good days and the bad, what to expect when you experience grief, how to communicate how you feel and a comprehensive support to understanding how to adjust you and your family to life without your loved one.

The New Normal is an adjustment, life is a completely different space now. But you are not alone. Self acceptance, adjustment and clarity is at hand.

Dedication

To my late husband Mick. At the time of writing it's been three years since you passed away, yet I know deep down you walk beside me every day. Together we created our beautiful family and we shared so many beautiful times together. You also taught me so much about grief, and that the world never stops. You taught me to keep moving forward.

Forever and deeply in my heart xx

Table of contents

vii	Dedication
ix	Table of contents
xi	Foreword
xiii	Acknowledgement
1	**CHAPTER 1 When grief hits you hard**
3	Heading home
4	Home
5	Grief theories
10	**CHAPTER 2 Before the funeral**
11	Common reactions to loss
12	Decision time!
15	Arranging the funeral
17	What to wear?
20	**CHAPTER 3 After the funeral**
21	Asking for help
22	Permit yourself to heal
22	Keep moving forward
23	What should you be doing now?
31	**CHAPTER 4 Looking after yourself**
32	What is self-care?
37	Journaling
38	Speak to people
39	Keep your thoughts in perspective
42	In memorium

46	**CHAPTER 5 Those special days**
51	Tips for dealing with milestones
56	**CHAPTER 6 When there are children involved**
57	Chloe was fourteen years old
58	Alex was fifteen years old
60	Jarred was twenty-five years old
62	Helping teens grieve
66	Helping 6 to 12-year-olds grieve
70	**CHAPTER 7 Myths and what the widow does not want to hear**
70	Common myths
77	What to say to a widow
78	General comforting words to say to someone who is grieving the loss of a loved one
78	One final word of advice when reaching out to a widow
80	**CHAPTER 8 Twelve months on. Now what?**
81	New normal. What does that even mean?
81	You need to be your cheerleader
82	Persistent complex bereavement disorder
83	Advice from my father
86	An ode to a widow
87	Bibliography
89	About the author
90	Testimonial

Foreword

Grief has touched our lives. My wonderful, warm and loving husband, passed in 2017. He touched the hearts of so many people in his life as a celebrated athlete and avid community supporter, but none so more than his family. I could not have dreamt of a better man to be my husband and the father of my children. Our family was always his number one priority for this incredible person.

The time and effort he put into parenting were as his dedication as an ironman. Dean and I adored each other and created a beautiful life together. He gave me four beautiful, amazing, kind boys — Brayden, Rory, Joshua and Lachlan. I'm so grateful to him for them.

We will miss him so much. His absence has left an unfilled hole in all our lives.

Grief can interrupt anyone's life in a single moment, and it is so incredibly important to know that you are supported on that journey and all its steps. I relate to Dr Olga's book so much, there is so much synergy with what I experienced and continue to experience as time passes. The strength a widow finds in herself is so evident in these pages. Dr. Olga's book will be the essential compassionate tool for the Widow as they step into the newness of an unexpected place that before now there was no guide. It is my pleasure to write this foreword, as I am now a part of a tribe and to be a part of the healing of those wounds for others is a legacy I embrace.

Yours in truth,
Reen Mercer

Acknowledgement

When I started writing this book, I knew that I could help other widows adjust to their New Normal. The book was my little secret, writing it became a process that provided time for me to reflect and grieve on my own. It allowed me to open up to grief as I wrote.

I would like to thank my two girls Alex and Chloe; you had to grow up quickly. Thank you for your support when I told you I was writing this book. I thank Jarred for his support and the three of you for your contributions to the book.

I shared my secret of writing this with two special friends, Jodi and Tanya. I thank them for their support now and after Mick passed away.

I thank Gary my partner, who has been understanding, supportive and given me the time I needed to write my book.

I would like to thank Shauna Blaak an Author and writer herself, thank you for your advice on writing. Thank you Maggie Wilde, my first Editor and Coach. You not only provided advice for the book, but you believed in me and believed I could do this. Thank you Kirsten Macdonald for the final edit and helping me design the book and get it ready to publish.

I thank family and friends who were there for my children and myself in our grief.

I would especially like to thank Mick's family for their ongoing support. We are truly blessed to continue to be close with you all.

My final thank you is to the two fathers' in my life. My own father for teaching me at a young age to be independent as you never know when adversity strikes. I thank my father-in-law Tony; I respect and am truly inspired by your strength. You shared with me how you coped after having lost a son in 1995, your wife, my mother-in-law Connie in 2013, and Mick seven months later

CHAPTER 1

When grief hits you hard

"People say you don't know what you've got until it's gone. The truth is, you know what you had; you just never thought you'd lose it."

~ Author Unknown

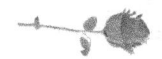

All I could hear was my staggered breathing between silent groans.

I needed air.

I needed to get out of there.

The room was spinning as the sounds of basketballs, and excited crowds faded into the distance. Darkness threatened to swallow me whole. I somehow managed to stumble down the seats and headed for the exit.

Don't fall.

I was vaguely aware of voices calling my name. "Olga, are you ok? What's wrong?"

"This can't be happening!" I heard myself say to no-one.

The cool air outside didn't help to relieve the pressure on my lungs. Panic, confusion. Where to go? What to do?

Oh, God. This nightmare has to be a dream. It can't be real. Not MY Mick.

All I could do is desperately remind myself "*Breathe, Olga, Breathe.*»

It's shocking how quickly 'life' can knock the wind out of you, isn't it? One minute I was enjoying my daughter's basketball game, and the next I was desperately trying not to faint from grief and shock.

Like most girls, I'd grown up with the dream of meeting that someone special, getting married, having children, watching them grow up, and then becoming grandparents. I knew what I wanted, and up until that moment, I was living my dream.

Little did I expect that a phone call from Mick's brother would deliver the devastating news that my husband of seventeen years had just died of a heart attack.

"What? MY Mick? No other Mick … MY Mick?"

"Yes," he said. "YOUR Mick."

I couldn't believe what I'd heard. Mick and his brother-in-law were only going to the race track at Moruya for the day. A three-hour drive from home. Their horse was scheduled to race, and then they were supposed to return. When Mick left, it wasn't meant to be the last time I said goodbye. Things like this happened to my clients, not me!

My mind recalled our wedding ceremony, seventeen years earlier. "… *to have and to hold, from this day forward, for better, for worse, for richer, for poorer, in sickness and in health, until death do us part.*"

Oh, God.

Never in my wildest nightmare did I expect the *"until death do us part"* to come so early. Suddenly, unexpectedly, he was gone. From the confusion of my loss, it was like a knife plunging into my heart, and I felt my world falling apart around me.

 Instantly I thought, What am I going to do? How am I going to tell the children?

The other parents who followed me outside now encircled me; deep concern etched on their faces. "What's wrong?" One by one, I just stared at them in shock and disbelief. My mouth wouldn't form words.

After minutes of silence and tears that ran in constant streams down my face, I managed to whisper, "My husband has just passed away." Now their faces looked like mine. Shock, disbelief, pain. Tears fell all around. Everyone was just as stunned as me.

I felt a sudden urgency to go home. Now. I needed to be in the place where we built our life together. I needed to feel his presence again.

"*Chloe and I need to go home.*"

The team manager went to fetch my daughter. She whispered into the coach's ear and then pulled her from the game. Some of the other mothers collected her bags, and they brought her outside to me.

Chloe was confused. She could tell that something bad had happened, but she had no idea what. I proceeded to tell her that her father had just "gone to heaven to be with Nonna," her grandmother who had died seven months before. We sat there crying together for a long time.

Then I remembered that my older daughter Alex was home alone. I was desperate to get to her; I didn't want anyone calling our house and telling her about her dad. She couldn't hear this terrible news from a stranger. I arranged instead for Mick's brother to go over to our house right away and break the news to her.

I said again, "We have to go home."

HEADING HOME

Thankfully, all the parents knew they needed to get me home as I wasn't in any state to drive. The trip home seemed like a lifetime. No clear thoughts were there, just my head spinning with questions upon questions "What am I going to do? What are we going to do? Oh, my gosh, what happened? How did it happen? What happened at the time? Where was he? I need to see him; I need to see him myself? How can I see him? I need answers…".

I turned to Chloe occasionally asking if she was okay? Her answers were always only a nod with her head and me saying "We will be okay." I rang our brother in law who was with Mick to get some answers; he said he was still with Mick, the ambulance, and police. He said he would ring me after and tell me everything, as he was also devastated, upset and trying to get his head around what happened. All I knew was that his body was going to Batemans Bay Hospital and I could not see him. I looked up at the sky, tears running down my face, hoping to see him one more time. Holding Chloe's hand, I thought *this does not make any sense.*

Then it dawned on me… is this what Mick meant when he said to me last week "under no circumstances can I change my plans on Saturday and take Chloe to basketball." I couldn't believe I never questioned Mick on that particular point; it was very unusual for him not to watch Chloe play. When I look back Mick made lots of little comments that didn't make sense in the week leading up to his death. Something inside me was stopping me saying *let him enjoy the week. I'll ask next Monday after Easter: what's with the strange comments all week?*

HOME

As we pulled up, a distraught Alex met us and the three of us hugged. We cried desperately; we tried to make sense of what was happening to us.

I went upstairs to our bedroom to be alone and sat for a long time on our bed. As I looked around at the familiar surroundings, the memories of our life flooded into my mind. Wave after wave, the events of our life together scrambled through my mind. Laughter, tears, highs, lows. Precious times together. Intimate times together. And I let the tears flow freely.

Then I went downstairs, replaying memorable moments with each room, each corner, each step. Vivid memories of our life together, perfectly synchronized like a Hallmark commercial. Still trying to make sense of it… it was surreal.

As I stood at the window looking out at the backyard, I remembered Mick always telling me,

> *"When your number's up, it's time to go. You don't have a choice. The world never stops. You have to keep going."*

Did Mick realize at the time that his words would burn inside me in the wake of his own death? I don't know. But what I did know was that, at this vulnerable moment, reeling from the emotional tsunami, I had a choice to make.

> **Was I going to sink or swim?**

Was I going to allow circumstances and debilitating grief to ruin my future and stop me from living? Or was I going to allow myself to feel the love and passion of a life well-lived, and walk through the process of grief with my girls, gracefully and successfully? Was I going to practice my own medicine?

I chose to swim. Mick's passing was a challenge that life had dealt me, and I was going to survive it to the best of my ability. I knew, somehow, I would find the resources within me to keep breathing. I was about to experience grief like many of my clients I helped. That's all I needed to do now.

So my journey began.

GRIEF THEORIES

I mentioned earlier that I am a Clinical Psychologist currently living in Australia. Over the course of my career, I've worked with many clients dealing with various forms and stages of grief.

But this was different. Now I was experiencing grief from the other side of the client/therapist relationship. I knew what was happening from a clinical perspective, but it's a whole different ball game when it happens to you.

Before we continue this journey through my story, importance must be placed on laying the groundwork for understanding grief and coping with grief.

There are many different theories that we use in the psychology industry concerning bereavement therapy. The main ones I've found particularly beneficial in my practice, and obviously more relevant after the death of my husband.

1. Stage theories

According to Elizabeth Kübler-Ross in her book called *Death and Dying*, there are five stages of grief. These are:
1. shock/denial,
2. anger/resentment/guilt,

3. bargaining,
4. depression, and
5. acceptance.

Her work was with dying patients has faced widespread criticism for suggesting that the grieving person must move through these five stages to successfully attain 'recovery' or 'closure.' The criticism lies mainly in the seductive promise of an 'emotional promised land' by oversimplifying a complicated process.

"*They [stage theories] are incapable of capturing the complexity, diversity and personal quality of the grieving experience. Stage models do not address the multiplicity of physical, psychological, social and spiritual needs encountered by the bereaved, their families and private networks.*"

In simpler terms, there is no formula for handling grief, everyone's experience is different.

Was I shocked? YES, but never in denial. I knew he was not coming back.

Was I angry, resentful and feel guilty? NO, NO and NO. What's the point, it won't bring him back, and it won't help me.

Did I bargain? NO, he was gone, I need to feel the pain. I can't control death.

Depression? NO, not clinically but yes feeling low in mood. I understood it was normal for me to feel down.

Acceptance? YES straight away! Life without Mick was my life now; I was a widow.

> *When I look back, I did not think about the stages at all. Nor did I experience all of them or did I experience them in any particular order.*

2. The dual process model of grief

This theory, developed in 1999 by Stroebe & Schut, describes grief as a process of moving between emotion-focused coping and problem-focused coping. With emotion-focused coping, the individual uses strategies to manage their negative emotional feelings. With problem-focused coping, a person focuses on the many external adjustments required by the loss and addresses the issues in the many ongoing life demands.

While being thrown into the depths of grief, I found that regardless of how I felt and in the depths of despair, I did not react to my emotions but responded to them, while at the same time slowly problem solved. I learned this through my study of psychology because managing my grief while at the same time emotionally supporting my children I needed to respond in a way that would help me achieve my goals. My goal of slowly moving forward step by step and taking each day as it comes. My goal of being able to continue to be the best mother I can to my children given my circumstances.

3. Task-based model

In his *Handbook for the Mental Health Practitioner*, J.W. Worden says that grieving is to be "considered as an active process that involves engagement with four tasks:

1. to accept the reality of the loss;
2. to process the pain of grief;
3. to adjust to a world without the deceased (including both internal, external and spiritual adjustments); and
4. to find an enduring connection with the deceased in the midst of embarking on a new life."

As time goes on, we continue to adjust to our life without our loved one. It's a lifetime journey of adjusting, one that never ends. I've always had a sixth sense, and I knew that in some way Mick would still be connected to us, and so he has in a way that only makes sense to me. When odd things would happen, or a close friend of ours would dream of seeing Mick and giving him messages to pass on to me. While some messages were clear others were cryptic that would only make sense later.

> *As time goes on, we continue to adjust to our life without our loved one. It's a lifetime journey of adjusting, one that never ends.*

4. Other factors that affect grieving

Some have also found that how we grieve is influenced by
1. Our ability to make sense of the loss,
2. The type of relationship one had with their spouse,
3. Finding a benefit such as growth in your character, and
4. The way the deceased died.

No marriage is perfect, and as I look back over the 17 years, we were like any normal married couple riding a rollercoaster full of ups and downs. But despite any challenges we had faced together or alone we were always there for each other, we supported each other in our goals and dreams and came through any hardships. I can honestly say Mick was an excellent husband, always wanting to provide for his family and wanting the best for us. He supported my career and helped with the kids and around the house.

Regardless of the theories, I threw them away and started to embrace and experience grief unlike any of my wildest nightmares.

> *This was my journey of grief, where are you on yours? Has this triggered anything for you? If you're reliving your grief you can always reach out for some help at my Facebook Group – Dr Olga's Widows Guide to Grief https://www.facebook.com/groups/widowsguidetogrief.*

As of 19 April 2014, I was a widow.

PROFESSIONAL NOTE

As a Clinical Psychologist, many of my clients suffering the loss of a loved one, regularly tell me they are not coping. I have found that many widows question the way they are grieving, they wonder what is normal, and many have not read anything on grief. I often hear other widows explain that they fear reading anything on grief, in case they discover they are not normal. By explaining to my clients,' the different models helps to normalize their reactions. It also helps them to stop fearing reading about grief. Professionally, I don't work from one model and use aspects from different models, because grief is not a one size fits all model.

CHAPTER 2

Before the funeral

"Grief is the price we pay for Love."

~ Queen Elizabeth II

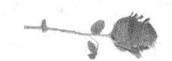

The morning after that dreadful day started earlier than I expected. There was no sunshine peeking through the curtains, and I didn't recall hearing the sound of my alarm clock, but I was definitely awake.

For a split second, I expected him to be waking up beside me, but then the reality of yesterday's events rolled over me again like a truck. Shock. Grief.

My husband was gone.

3:00 am?

Part of me wanted to will myself back to sleep, to that in-between place where I could still hear his voice and feel his touch. Even then, I could still smell the scent of his skin on the pillow beside me. This CAN'T be happening.

But I was a clinical psychologist, a professional. I knew that no amount of imagination would change the reality of this new life of mine. There was no point in railing at the heavens and demanding to know "why?" Logically, I knew there was no point in going around in circles and driving myself insane.

As I threw back the covers, I heard his voice again in my mind,

When your number's up, it's time to go. You don't have a choice. The world never stops. You have to keep going.

He was right, of course. We don't get to control these things; they just happen. I took a deep breath and let it out slowly. I faced a life without my husband… it slowly dawned on me this was my new reality.

Let's talk for a few minutes about "What is normal?"

If your world has just come crashing down, and you've lost someone incredibly dear to you. What should you be feeling right now?

From both personal and my professional opinion, here are some common reactions that people often experience following a significant loss. You may experience all of them, some of them, or none of them at all. You may experience them right away, or months down the road. Just know that these reactions are normal. So, wherever you're at now, it's crucial to know that you are normal.

Please understand… there is no right or wrong way to grieve.

COMMON REACTIONS TO LOSS

Emotional Reactions: Sadness, shock, anger, guilt, jealousy, anxiety, fear, shame, relief, feeling powerless, hopeless or helpless, feeling irritable and frustrated, loneliness, yearning/longing.

Upon hearing the news of Mick's death, I was in shock; I just could not believe it. It was unexpected and sudden. During that first week, there was sadness, anxiety, and fear about the future, a strong sense of feeling alone and yearning and longing to see and speak to him just one more time. The 'busyness' of preparing for the funeral and thoughts rushing through my mind also led to feeling irritable.

Over time, anxiety has come at different times, and I am less fearful about my future. I never felt hopeless or helpless because I still knew that somehow, I would be able to deal with things/problems/issues as they arise. I felt lonely at home for a long time, the warmth of home suddenly left me as well, until we moved house, to somewhere smaller.

Physical Reactions: headaches, nausea, tiredness, loss of appetite, insomnia, sensitivity to various stimuli, in particular, noise, muscular tension, exhaustion, pain, lack of energy, tightness in chest, shortness of breath

I had headaches, felt tired and had no appetite. I always felt tense and did not sleep well waking early at 3 am.

I remember one morning having a pounding headache, like someone hitting me with a hammer repeatedly on my head headache. It just wouldn't go away no matter what sort of pain relief I took. As I was talking to Mick's son Jarred in the kitchen while in the throes of the pain in my head I suddenly said, "I feel sick, I need to vomit." Within seconds, I started to be physically ill.

Cognitive Reactions: disbelief, denial, obsessive thinking, apathy, numbness. Not being able to concentrate or remember. Looping thought patterns and continuous what if scenarios. Disorientation, confusion, lack of motivation, impaired judgment, depression, lack of control, resentment, wanting to find a culprit to ease the pain, wanting to damage something to ease the pain, dreaming, diminished self concern, emptiness, replaying images of loss

My initial reaction was one of disbelief about what I was hearing, I became numb and felt confused … confused about what to do, there were just no logical thoughts. All of a sudden, I felt empty. The week leading up to the funeral I went into an automatic pilot mode, doing what was necessary for Mick to have a sweet farewell, thinking what he would like. For other things, I was unmotivated. That feeling of being unmotivated persisted, for some months, but despite the feeling, I continued to do what was necessary.

While I had some of these emotional, physical, and cognitive reactions, I knew that it was okay to feel like this.

What about you?

Has this triggered anything for you?

Are you starting to feel these emotions again?

If you answered yes and you need some help, join me for support on my Facebook Group – Dr Olga's Widows Guide to Grief https://www.facebook.com/groups/widowsguidetogrief.

DECISION TIME!

I remember that first morning, as I sat in the silent house with my morning coffee, it dawned on me that I had some MAJOR DECISIONS to make.

More than just what to wear at the funeral, or what food to serve to visitors, I had to decide how I was going to survive.

1. Would I sink or swim?

Sitting, staring blankly out the window I thought to myself *"Oh my gosh how will we survive, how will I survive?"* The answer to these questions may seem obvious, but I assure you, it's not. Many people never recover from a traumatic loss. Why else do you think trauma affects relationships or so many people struggle for years to make sense of what happened?

I was a mother of two teenage girls and to a 26-year-old son from Mick's previous relationship. I didn't have the luxury of crawling under a rock and hiding. It was my responsibility as a mother to pull my children, through this, especially my two young teenage girls, to drag them along with me, and to care for them in their grief.

2. How will the kids cope?

I chose to not fall apart for my kids' sakes. I consciously decided to be there emotionally for them as they came to terms with losing their father. While children can undoubtedly be supportive, and they were, it wasn't their responsibility to care for me in my grief. **It was my job to care for them in their grief.**

> *While children can undoubtedly be supportive, and they were, it wasn't their responsibility to care for me in my grief.* **It was my job to care for them in their grief.**

I also chose not to be angry. Yes, I know that anger is a natural and normal reaction to loss, but it serves no purpose. Anger wasn't going to help anyone, least of all the grieving widow and her children.

During this time, I found that my emotions were reasonably stable while everyone was around me and we were busy preparing for the funeral. However, it was once family and friends went home that the real loneliness hit. It was in those moments that I had to remind myself that Mick wasn't coming back It was in those moments, even though I didn't know how to 'swim' in my new reality, that I still chose to swim.

I enjoyed the silence of the quiet house as I contemplated this strange new world around me. I recalled, my coffee cup was empty, and my silence was abruptly interrupted with family and friends arriving, and the phone always ringing.

Contemplating my strange new life without Mick led me to another critical decision-making moment…

3. Was I going to accept help?

Even as I write this, I remember being shocked at how incredibly busy I was in the role of *"the widow planning the funeral,"* now my new marital status. "A widow," I thought to myself. It was strange to call myself a widow now. Something that I would expect from a woman much older than me.

I never expected that level of busyness. Ever.

People came over every day, all shocked by what happened. And given what Mick believed, *"The world never stops. You have to keep going,"* I felt I had to support them through their shock. How odd is that, I remember thinking *"I was the widow supporting everybody else."* It was exhausting.

I remember Mick telling me several times over the years that if he died first, he didn't want everyone to be sad. He wanted us to celebrate the life he had and everything he had achieved.

> *He insisted "I don't want a wake that's sad. I want a party that celebrates my life!"*

I found it so interesting that, while he was alive, Mick never wanted me to throw him a party… ever. But for his wake, he did.

You may be asking yourself right now, "When did I get time just to cry or comfort myself?"

The answer was, "Before people arrive and after people leave."

My advice to you during this incredibly busy and stressful time is to PLEASE ACCEPT HELP FROM FAMILY AND FRIENDS! I know you probably like to do things a certain way, and you want everything to be 'perfect,' but you have other more important things to attend to, such as:

- You need to grieve and make sense of your new world.
- You need to comfort your children as they try to make sense of their world now.
- You need to attend to the funeral arrangements.

Even though I was quite independent, I permitted myself to delegate tasks to others to help us and provide the support I needed.

4. Was I going to allow myself to laugh again?

I realize that you may feel like you're drowning in waves of sadness right now, allow yourself to take time to 'look for the laughter' in the middle of the grief.

Even during my deepest sorrow, there was also much laughter, and it was laughter that strengthened me to move to the next step.

While family and friends were over, we spent a lot of time talking about Mick. There were so many memories to share. We remembered his sayings and the funny things he had done throughout his life. During that time it felt so good to laugh, it was so therapeutic.

It's so important in the early days of grief to NOT stop the laughter when it comes. It's good for you to celebrate the life lived. While laughing, I was confident that Mick knew we were celebrating his life. And as I pictured the grin on Mick's face, I knew that he was laughing with us too.

 It's so important in the early days of grief to NOT stop the laughter when it comes. It's good for you to celebrate the life lived.

ARRANGING THE FUNERAL

The funeral is crucial to the emotional healing of all those left behind. Whether you choose to have a funeral, memorial, wake, or something else altogether, this event is the farewell for the deceased, an opportunity for all family members, friends, and acquaintances to say goodbye.

For me, Mick was not just a loving husband and father; he was also a son, a brother, a brother-in-law, and an uncle. Therefore, we all planned his funeral.

By 'we,' I mean his father, brothers, sister, brother-in-law, and sister-in-law. It was important to all of us. This was their loss as well as mine, and planning the funeral together with me would allow them to help lay him to rest too.

While planning the funeral, it's important to consider more than just what you want, but also **what your loved one liked** and **if they didn't leave a plan what they may have wanted**. You'd be surprised how many people don't discuss these matters at all before something like this happens. Perhaps, they feel the topic particularly morbid, or uncomfortable, or even bad luck. Either way, such discussions are necessary and incredibly helpful, and I would highly encourage you to discuss these matters with your loved ones while there is still time. Give attention to details such as:

- What to expect should one, or both of you die.
- Do you both know the details of life insurance, the Will, and other financial matters?
- Do you know each other's likes and preferences for a funeral/memorial/wake?

I never expected to be a widow in the prime of my life having to make arrangements about what Mick would have wanted… but it happened. Thankfully, Mick and I had that discussion in advance, so I knew what he liked and what he wanted.

Busyness

A friend recently asked me what my strongest memory was at this time. My answer was, "Oh my God, the busyness! You don't get to breathe."

As a new widow planning a funeral keeps you busy with hundreds of things to decide, including:

- Choosing the content and design of the memorial book.
- Finding suitable photos of your loved one to do justice to their life.
- Meeting with the priest/clergy/funeral celebrant to discuss the funeral.
- Choosing the wording for the obituary in the newspaper.
- Considering likes and preferences of your loved one concerning their funeral.

While Funeral Directors organize the funeral, you still need to make so many decisions yourself.

> *I kept the children informed of what the plans for the funeral were and involved them in much of the process that I could. They participated in choosing photos of their father and helping with the content and design of the memorial book. This way they were involved in laying their father to rest.*

WHAT TO WEAR?

Another important task is to decide what you and the children are going to wear. Let's be realistic; it's not as if you have been saving that one dress for your husband's funeral. So, out you go into the big, wide world to shop for something to wear.

My advice… take someone with you, because you don't need to do this alone. I went with my sister-in-law. Even still, it felt as if the world was spinning while I stood there in a daze. I felt alone, and I was unsure where even to start choosing an outfit. Familiarity was necessary, so I went to my favourite shop, and I just sat down while the manager picked several dresses for me to try on.

I always dressed well and had my hair done when Mick and I would go out together. I did the same for his farewell. I put my make-up on and was ready to embrace all the negative feelings associated with grief and laying my loving husband to rest.

Here is my best piece of advice yet…

Have a private viewing before the family gets there.
When someone dies, it's my family custom to have a viewing the day before the funeral. While Jarred came as well, my girls did not. They said they did not want to see their father in a coffin, and that was okay. I wanted them to remember their last image of him being alive.

I remember that day; I couldn't wait to go and see Mick I ached to finally be with him and be able to say everything I needed to say to him. I wanted to talk about my shock and surprise at what had happened, about my fears for the future, and that I understood what I needed to do. How did I know? Mick and I had discussed what we would do as a couple if he or I should ever die. I didn't like it, but I'm glad we did. I knew what to do.

You have to keep going.
As I walked into the viewing to see him for the first time, I was aching, nervous and excited, all at the same time, and then just burst into tears, pouring down my face. Having Mick all to myself was wonderful. However, I instantly noticed that they didn't do his hair properly and I told him so. I also said not to worry and that I'd fix him up, and then I started styling his hair the way he liked it.

I spent an hour with Mick and said everything I wanted to. I was able to give him a personal letter which may not have made sense to anyone else, but it didn't matter; it was from my heart, and I remember it being a beautiful, private, intimate moment.

To this day, this private time with my husband remains the highlight of the whole ordeal. I'm so grateful for the time I had with him. It was a lovely moment to an incredibly difficult week.

As I left the viewing, I felt the apprehension in my heart. The funeral was tomorrow, and it will be my chance to say goodbye to Mick with my family. I didn't want to think about it, but the thoughts kept coming.
- How can I say goodbye forever?
- How will I cope tomorrow?
- Oh, my gosh, I'll lay him to rest, and then what happens the day after?

I knew that I needed to rest so I could handle what would come tomorrow. I remember as I lay my head on my pillow I prayed and hoped that sleep would come easily.

PROFESSIONAL NOTE
Having a viewing lessens the likelihood of denial and disbelief, especially if the death is unexpected and sudden. If you choose not to have a viewing or have been advised not to, you can have one in your mind. Or another option is to have your own time with a photo of your loved one and some other special belongings of your loved one. You can write a letter to them and choose afterward what you do with that letter, for example, bury it with them or have it cremated with them. It's up to you what you do with it. If children attend a viewing, inform them previously of what to expect. Many children cope better than adults expect. It also helps them to process their grief.

CHAPTER 3

After the funeral

"Grief is like the ocean; it comes on waves ebbing and flowing. Sometimes the water is calm, and sometimes it is overwhelming. All we can do is learn to swim."

~ Vicki Harrison

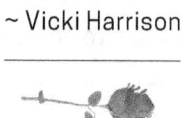

In the weeks following the funeral, I remember how exhausted I felt, both physically and emotionally. The busyness that had overwhelmed me before the funeral was mostly over, family and friends had gone home, and I found myself alone, more alone than ever, lost in my little corner of the world.

Understanding the loneliness

Have you ever wondered why many people don't visit or ring after a funeral?

It's vital to remember that everyone grieves differently. Some people stay away because they want to give you privacy. That's not a bad thing. Despite feeling anxious and fearful, you need time to process what has just happened to you.

Other people stay away because they just don't know what to say or do to help you feel better. Perhaps that's because they haven't walked through it themselves, or maybe their memories are too fresh to share. Either way, nothing they do or say at this point will make you feel better. This is your time to grieve. Only by letting out your emotions will you begin to heal.

I remember the day after the funeral so clearly. Friends who stayed the night left to go home. I felt a sense of relief to be on my own to shut myself away from the outside world. To not have to talk but be alone in my pain, pain that no one could take away. As the days went on over that first week time alone was precious to me. It allowed me to let my negative emotions come and go, cry when I wanted to, do nothing when I wanted to. I needed this time to feel the loneliness despite the children being home. I needed to allow my thoughts to flow freely. Those thoughts *"What do I do now?" "What should I do?" "I'm so tired" "How will the kids cope?"* on and on they went with no answers.

I knew it was normal to have questions run through my mind and no answers. I also knew that it was important not to make any life-changing decisions that I may regret later. I relied on having time to think things through and eventually have the answers come to me.

ASKING FOR HELP

On the other hand, there are others who worry about you being alone, and they want to spend time with you. Their intentions come from their heart, and they're only doing what they think is right.

But if you find yourself wanting time alone, then you're going to have to find a way to tell them *what you want* and *what you need* politely.

For example,

1. If you want to be alone, kindly explain that you need to be alone, and let them know that you'll ring them if you need company. Or you can ask them to contact you in a few days.
2. Likewise, if you want people around, then call your family or friends and ASK them to visit.

Unfortunately, people can't read your mind, despite the fact that they love you. Communicate clearly during this time, rather than expecting people to know what you want and then later being angry at them which could potentially damage a valuable relationship.

You will find that people will appreciate knowing what you want and what your needs are.

While close friends rang to check how I was managing, I also spoke regularly to the family. I didn't mind being alone as it gave me a chance to go through Mick's things. Spend time thinking about our life together over the past 17 years.

PERMIT YOURSELF TO HEAL

During this period, I was left alone with my thoughts and my memories, but I didn't mind. I wanted time alone so that I could work out what I needed to do. I also wanted time to allow myself to feel the pain of separation, the ache in my heart, the fear, the anxiety, and to cry.

Crying is part of the healing process. Sitting with these emotions and allowing myself to 'feel' them lessened the pain each day.

Yes, there was a lot of pain. Yes, despite the sun shining and other people being happy, the world seemed dull and grey. Yes, there were moments that I wanted to close myself off from the outside world. But I couldn't escape the memory of Mick saying to me, *"The world keeps going,"* and I knew that I had to keep going too.

I remember going to bed each night and crying, then all of a sudden warmth would envelop my body, and I would suddenly stop crying, feel calm and peaceful. It was as if Mick came and hugged me and let me know that everything would be okay. It was an odd experience, but one that gave me comfort.

KEEP MOVING FORWARD

Have you noticed that the world hasn't stopped? The temptation for every grieving person is to stop and hide, but the world will continue moving. Suddenly, household bills will arrive, and if you don't keep moving forward, it will be too hard to catch up later.

Yes, I know that things are overwhelming now, but imagine how much more overwhelming they will be if you completely do nothing.

Now is the time to take small steps to *'walk your marathon.'* The steps don't have to be big, and you don't have to run. Just keep moving. Doing little things one-at-a-time will keep you from feeling even more overwhelmed later. Remember if all becomes too much you can join me for support on my Facebook Group – Dr Olga's Widows Guide to Grief https://www.facebook.com/groups/widowsguidetogrief.

Now is the time to take small steps to 'walk your marathon.'

Having to go to the letterbox to check the post gave me a feeling of dread. Why? It meant that I had to connect to the outside world. There was a genuine fear that I would see his name on letters as if nothing had happened. It was another reminder that I was all alone, anxious about everything I needed to do. I didn't like that the mail showed me that the world hadn't stopped, it was like no one cared that I was a grieving widow and people just wanted their money! Was this maybe my anger in grief? Angry that the world wouldn't stop for me to have a rest and try to work things out?

WHAT SHOULD YOU BE DOING NOW?
Contact all relevant parties
Depending on how busy your local government offices are, it could take anywhere from two to seven weeks to receive a copy of the death certificate. Without the document itself, you cannot finalize certain necessary tasks. For example, you will not be able to complete changes to your banking information until the bank receives a copy of the death certificate.

However, there are still a lot of things that you can do while waiting. The best thing to do is to make a list of what needs to be done and tick each item as you complete it.

Below is a checklist of some organizations and people that you need to notify of the death of your loved one. This is not an exhaustive list; you are welcome to add or delete any items to make it relevant to your situation.

Organisations/persons to be notified of death
- Solicitor, lawyer
- Taxation Office

- Electoral Commission
- Public Health Care Institutions (i.e. Medicare)
- Private Health Insurance
- Social Welfare Organizations (i.e. Centrelink, Social Security department, etc.)
- Child support services
- Banking Institutions
- Insurance companies
- Superannuation fund
- Schools
- Telecommunications providers (e.g. phone and internet)
- Utilities (e.g. gas and electricity)
- Vehicle registration and licensing authority
- Clubs
- Health Professionals (e.g. doctor, dentist, optometrist, podiatrist, physiotherapists)
- Unions
- Social and sports clubs
- _____
- _____
- _____

If you'd like to download this list, you can join me at <u>Dr Olga's Widows Guide to Grief Support Group</u> https://www.facebook.com/groups/widowsguidetogrief.

Notifying organizations and people can be tiresome and emotionally draining. You may feel desperate to finish the task as soon as possible, do remember that some things take time. So, don't panic or fret. Just breathe and take it one-day-at-a-time.

I remember going to the bank to let them know Mick passed away. As I was walking with his death certificate in my hand, my eyes welled up with tears, and I couldn't hold them back. I didn't care because I was a grieving widow, and I didn't care that people would see me crying in public. I didn't care what they thought, because how do you hold back tears when you're in emotional pain. I had my list of organizations to notify. So, I crossed each one off as I slowly completed my list with or without tears. I was surprised that contacting some of these organizations I felt fine, and then all of a sudden grief would hit me, and I felt overwhelmed. I just focused on one at a time.

Sorting out our loved one's things

The first few weeks alone gave me a chance to go through all of Mick's things. It's a difficult task that some people avoid for years, refusing to let go of the past. But I remember thinking

> *Why keep his clothes? I know that he's not coming back, no matter how badly I hurt.*

So, I used this time to sort through his wardrobe, saying 'goodbye' one item at a time, and keeping only his favourite t-shirt and personal things that were important to him. I also took the opportunity to give things to all three children; I made sure it was equal between them. This process of sorting through Mick's things allowed me to keep saying goodbye and move steadily forward while still keeping him close to my heart.

> *Everybody is different, and while some people want to hold onto their loved one's things longer, others sort through their possessions sooner. There is no right or wrong with this and you the widow will know when the time is okay for you.*

Making decisions

Throughout these first few weeks, as I sorted through memories and continued my journey through grief, the thought kept going through my mind… *"Now what?"* The girls were quite anxious how we would survive financially, no matter how much I told them we'd be okay, they said they would get casual jobs after school to help me pay the bills.

Thankfully, I was able to take three weeks off from work, but I had clients and responsibilities that needed my attention. I couldn't afford to hide in my house for months on end. Yes, the world was grey, and the food was tasteless, but I had to keep going.

As a mother, I also needed to help my children get back into a routine. Mick had passed away during the Easter holiday, so thankfully we were able to rest for a bit. Jarred went on with his day to day activities, and the girls were eager to get back to their friends and regular school routine, and I didn't blame them.

Here are some practical things to consider, especially as a mother, as you make decisions concerning your new reality:

1. Your new routine
   - What can you ask your children to help you with at home?
   - What new chores can you allocate to them?
2. Your budget
   - Have you looked at your budget?
   - How will you organize it and know when each of your bills is due?
3. When will you go back to work?
   - Do you have customers/clients/staff/bosses that are depending on you?
   - Do you need to work to meet your financial responsibilities?
4. What help will you need with the children?
   - Who will transport them to and from school, or to out-of-school activities?
   - Who will help your children before and after school?
   - Who will be with them if you need to go out in the evenings?
5. What other things will you need help with, and who will you ask?
   - House maintenance?

- Gardens?
- Car maintenance?

And while this is not a time to be making any major life decisions, realistically, it may be a chance to start thinking about your future and what your options are. Should you stay where you're living now, or would moving be a better choice? Can you afford it? Can you handle the upkeep of your current house, or would a smaller place be more manageable?

For me, I needed to make the important decision of what to do. It was a decision that was not hard to make because realistically, as a single mother having to work full-time, *how was I going to maintain a large house, financially afford all the bills, and support financially two young girls?*

I've always claimed I'm a realist so despite the emotional turmoil I was in, logically I knew what I needed to do.

Only listen to good advice
When you start thinking about your future, you will find that a lot of people will be giving you advice; some of it you will ask for, and some of it will be just voluntary. And some people may even be shocked by your decisions.

It's important to remember that,

This is YOUR life, and no one else is walking in your shoes.
What may be right for them may not be right for you. You need to base your decisions on what you can manage, and what can help you. Even your children will be okay with your decisions when made confidently and with their best interests at heart.

There were a lot of people wondering what I was going to do now that Mick was gone. One thing he always said was,

Don't listen to other people. Who cares what they say.
Those were words that I took to heart because this new time in my life was about ME. It had to be. I was a widow raising young teenage girls, and I also

needed to work full-time. I needed to make decisions that would empower me to do both well.

Some people may find this attitude selfish, but it's not selfish at all. The widow needs to put herself first because if she doesn't look after herself, she won't be able to care for the children. I realized that the girls were getting older, Jarred was an adult and that, one day in the not-too-distant future, they would move out and I'd be on my own. I needed to live somewhere where I could manage on my own and not be a burden on them.

> *Some people may find this attitude selfish, but it's not selfish at all. The widow needs to put herself first because if she doesn't look after herself, she won't be able to care for the children.*

Mick's brother and sister also spoke to me about thinking about moving to an apartment closer to them all. Something that I could financially afford and for us to feel safe. While I could not financially afford a four-bedroom apartment, they offered for Jarred to live with his grandfather.

For that reason, four months later, I decided to sell our home. The house was too big and needed too much work to keep up. **"A house is only brick and mortar, but your memories are always with you,"** a family friend told me. You won't lose them; you'll take them anywhere you go. Besides this, a move into an apartment was a long-term plan Mick, and I had together.

Yes, I received criticism for my decision, but those people weren't walking in my footsteps. Nor were they in previous discussions with my husband when we discussed what I should do in such a circumstance. I knew what Mick would say, and that's all I needed. I knew what I had to do, and I grew in strength with each decision as his words kept repeating in my mind, **"Don't listen to other people."**

Eight months after his death, we moved, the girls and I moved into a smaller place that was within walking distance to work and the beach. The girls were very keen to go because they could not cope living in the house anymore, knowing their father was not coming home. They also saw the stress the house put on me trying to manage it on my own. They always said to me "it will get better Mum once we move, we'll start again, it will be easier for you." It was the right decision for all of us, and our quality of life improved significantly.

While some Widows remain living in their house, especially those with young children, others have moved. What's right for some may not be right for others. Each situation is unique, and therefore there is no right or wrong.

This was the start of our new normal, and I've also shared a little story about Jenny that may help you too.

CASE STUDY

Jenny was a 45-year-old widow with two teenage children. She came to see me three months after her husband's death because she felt she was not coping, was not sleeping well, and was very anxious. She had still not returned to work. Her husband always took care of the bills and budgeted for the family. Jenny had not been able to decide what to do because she was frightened of making the wrong decisions. Part of Jenny's treatment was problem-solving to look at her current situation, her options financially and how she would manage daily now and in the future. She started to write everything down that she needed to decide on and categorized everything into groups: managing financially, managing her time and children's needs, working out a new routine. By writing things down and looking at various solutions, she started to gain some sense of control over her current life. She had learned there are no guarantees that any decision made is right until you start to act on that decision to see if it works. If not, decisions can be amended. By making the smaller minor decisions first, and major decisions later when you could cope with your grief, Jenny slowly learned that some of her anxiety focused on worrying about what to do. She learned that decisions need to be logical and practical not solely based on how she felt at the time.

When we left our home, I had a final goodbye on my own. It wasn't the house that made the memories; it was our life together. And we've never looked back. While Jarred lives with his grandfather, he comes over once a week for dinner and we're still together at other significant events. We are still family.

CHAPTER 4

Looking after yourself

"I have come to believe
that caring for myself is not self-indulgent.
Caring for myself is an act of survival."

~ Audre Lorde

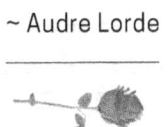

As the weeks went by and the pain in my heart continued, I discovered that there is no sound so irritating as an alarm clock, and no sight so painful as sunlight. In these circumstances these sensitivities are normal.

It's okay to want to stay asleep, trying desperately to find that in-between place where your loved one is still sleeping beside you.

It's normal to be irritated by the sunshine why should other people's world continue to spin when mine has completely crashed?

Cringing at the sounds of laughter and loud conversation is normal, *why should they be happy when I'm dying inside?*

It's no wonder that many widows feel overwhelmed after their loved ones have died.

But, you cannot stay in this surreal place between living and not-living, especially if you have children who are depending on you. They too are suffering from their own grief, and you cannot afford to stay in bed with the blinds shut.

I understand that you don't know what to do and the simplest decisions seem impossible, but IT'S TIME FOR SELF-CARE.

If you are struggling with caring for yourself during your grief, help is available. Join me for support on my Facebook Group – Dr Olga's Widows Guide to Grief hhttps://www.facebook.com/groups/widowsguidetogrief

WHAT IS SELF-CARE?

Self-care is taking action to care for yourself at this critical time – to do what is required to care for your physical needs, emotional and also mental needs. For example, taking time out for yourself, having a relaxing bath, having a massage, preparing healthy food to support your body and cells as you grieve, go for a walk, taking time out to talk to someone you trust who will listen rather than tell you what to do.

> *Self-care is taking action to care for yourself at this critical time – to do what is required to care for your physical needs, emotional and also mental needs.*

Why is self-care so important? Because being responsible and looking after yourself is important during your journey. For example, if you stop putting fuel in your car or servicing it, one day it won't be able to meet you or your family's needs. Therefore, self-care is putting the fuel you need in your tank to meet your needs and those of your children. It will help you to care for your kids, as they need you more than ever now.

"I remember thinking I did not choose to be a widow or a single parent, but that is what life dealt me. I knew I needed to look after myself so I could maintain physical and emotional strength to care for my kids. I needed to show them that, despite the tragedy that occurred around us, looking after ourselves is important. I needed to show them how to keep going."

Here are some areas of self-care that you can apply today.

I did not choose to be a widow or a single parent, but that is what life dealt me. I knew I needed to look after myself so I could maintain physical and emotional strength to care for my kids.

Eat healthy

While eating healthy is always important, it is especially important when you're grieving. Grief puts a lot of strain on the body, and we need to eat healthy so we can nourish ourselves to combat those stresses. Yes, I understand

that you have no appetite and that food has no flavor, but you still need to eat to fuel your body.
- Try eating smaller meals throughout the day to supply the energy you need to deal with everyday life.
- Drink plenty of water! It's imperative that you keep yourself hydrated.
- Avoid any alcohol or drugs. You only gain temporary relief, and you'll feel worse afterward. Negative emotions will be even harder to deal with under the adverse effects of alcohol.

It's strange how grief makes you forget how to cook, and takes away any desire to do grocery shopping. In my deepest pain, eating and shopping were not on the top of my daily agenda.

For years, I had faithfully made the girls' lunches for school, but after Mick died, I couldn't do it anymore. It was like I was completely uninspired and didn't know where to start. Initially, I gave them money to buy food at school, but after a week I remember them saying to me, "Can we go grocery shopping and make lunches again? We'll help you."

I then knew it was time to start the weekly task of grocery shopping and making lunches. I told them, "I will try my best to make lunch for school." Notice I used the word "try"? I did that because I knew that I'd be hard on myself if I missed a day, and I didn't want to set myself up for failure. **Try to resume your normal duties and acknowledge you're doing the best you can.**

Let others know they can help

Family and friends always ask how they can help. Let them know what they can do for you; you're not alone. For example, request people to make casseroles or other healthy dishes that you can freeze.

While I didn't have to ask for people to make healthy meals for me, there were plenty of meals delivered ready to be put in the freezer. I remember one friend asked my sister in law before visiting what could she bring. She arrived with a fruit and vegetable hamper. I thought to myself *"how wonderful is this."* I never really asked for help until my journey with grief. I knew it was okay to do this. I had family and friends help with grocery shopping, laundry, and general cleaning.

Start some exercise

No, I'm not pressuring you to run a marathon or join a fancy gym. I know you don't have the energy for that right now, and having to start something new is the *last* thing on your mind.

What I'm suggesting isn't about exercising 'full-speed-ahead,' but rather about doing SOMETHING.

- It's about **physical health**, going outside and getting back to some form of physical activity is good for you. Don't wait for motivation; just do it.
- Think of the smell of fresh air around you, the warmth of the sun on your body, your thoughts drifting into the sky above, and each step you take is a move in the direction of seeing yourself more positively. Think about how you'll feel after being in the fresh air, the clear mind and feeling more refreshed. Use this brain training trick to create more energy and motivation to get outside.
- It's also about **mental health**, you can't stay in your house forever. Even going outside for a short walk will help to clear your mind and get some much-needed Vitamin D.

Get a check up

As with many forms of trauma, the stress of grief can wear you down physically. As such, it is important to get a full physical check-up from your doctor especially with existing medical conditions that might be negatively impacted by grief.

Yes, I realize that doctors or hospitals may be frightening right now, especially if they were part of the journey of your grief, but choose to do it for you and your children. Check-ups are a part of life. Don't give into fear. You are the ONLY parent your kids have, and taking care of your health is the responsible thing to do for you and them.

I remember experiencing chest pain soon after Mick's death. My immediate thought was, *"Oh, no! I'm going to die from a heart attack too."* After a few days, I went to the doctor and explained my symptoms. I told them about Mick and said, "I need to know if this is anxiety or not. I've never felt this before."

I'm so glad that I went because, after an urgent ECG and blood test, we discovered that it was neither a heart attack nor a panic attack… I had a chest infection. All the more reason to take action on self-care. Your immune system will be reacting to the stress you're experiencing emotionally. If I'd not gone to the doctor things may have worsened.

Allow yourself to feel

Let me bring your attention back to the quote at the beginning of Chapter 3.

> *"Grief is like the ocean; it comes on waves ebbing and flowing. Sometimes the water is calm, and sometimes it is overwhelming. All we can do is learn to swim." - Vicki Harrison*

That is such an excellent description of grief. Grief is a process, an ongoing process that continues even when you start looking after yourself. There is no 'quick-fix.' **There will still be many times when waves of emotion will roll over you with force.** When this happens, acknowledge and be mindful of those times.

Grief is a process, an ongoing process that continues even when you start looking after yourself.

Say to yourself:
- I am feeling angry…
- I am feeling sad…
- I am feeling a sharp pain in my heart…
- I am feeling anxious…

Allow yourself to feel those things and don't judge them to be right or wrong, good or bad. They are normal right now.

Notice which physical sensations accompany your emotions. For example,
- When you feel pain in your heart, say to yourself, "I'm curious that I am leaning forward with my hand on my heart."
- With anger, say "I notice that I've tensed up, and have clenched my jaw."

You can also do this when you feel moments of relief, happiness, or another pleasant feeling you have.
- For example, "I feel happy, and I notice that I have a smile on my face."

> *Feelings can change from minute-to-minute, hour-to-hour, and day-to-day. Allow yourself to sit with your feelings and don't avoid them. They are yours, and yours alone, and there is no right or wrong way to feel. Avoiding negative emotions will only make them return stronger than before.*

Remember, they are only feelings. They are your way of processing typical emotional reaction to grief. They cannot hurt you. What hurts you is your fear, avoidance, and reactions to negative emotions. So rather than avoiding them, allow yourself to breathe and feel everything. You will notice that the negative emotions will soon pass, witness them with curiosity each time they come, you'll see the intensity will eventually lessen.

As a Clinical Psychologist, I knew about the art of mindfulness and being 'in the moment.' It was my time to sit with my negative emotions, and fully feel and experience them. I needed to feel the grief, allow myself to cry, and acknowledge that what I'm feeling is normal. As time went on, I noticed that the intensity decreased and my feelings resolved themselves sooner. And while those negative emotions physically drained me, I knew this was my time to nurture and self-soothe.

I knew this was my time to nurture and self-soothe.

Be kind to yourself

Negative feelings are normal during grief when you are in the middle of the storm; do not to allow your negative feelings to stop you from looking after yourself. I know that you don't 'feel' like pampering yourself. I know that you don't 'feel' like having fun. That's ok. Where you're at now is part of your soul health, it is part of your strategy for survival.

Pampering yourself and doing things that you used to enjoy won't instantly improve how you feel. But over time, regular self-care will help you cope with your negative feelings, and you'll find your mood improving. Everyone's reaction will be different, but it starts with asking yourself, *"What did I once enjoy?"*
- Relaxing in a candlelit bath.
- Giving yourself a facial, pedicure, manicure, etc.
- Listening to your favourite music.
- Meeting up with friends and family.

If you have to at first, see it as re-fuelling the engine that is your body. One day, you will wake up to discover that the world is not so grey anymore, but has colour again.

I remember looking at photos of our wedding and feeling the tears pouring down my face. I would spend hours looking at our photo albums and reminiscing our times together: when we had the kids, our holidays, and when we went out with friends and family. There were lots of tears (as well as smiles) remembering the happy times, I'd even find myself laughing (despite the darkness) when I remembered funny things he used to do and say.

Afterwards, I would have a good cry, and then pamper myself with a long hot shower to wash the tears away.

JOURNALING

Grief tends to overwhelm us with waves of negative thoughts and emotions. Sometimes we do a decent job of holding that negativity inside with thoughts spinning in our minds.

My best advice to you, even if you've never done so before, is KEEP A JOURNAL.

Journaling is about getting your thoughts and feelings OUT onto paper and finding clarity. You don't have to be eloquent or coherent, and you certainly don't have to be a poet. No one is grading you on spelling and grammar, and you can destroy the pages later if you don't want anyone to see them. This technique helps you find a voice for your pain.

> *Journaling is about getting your thoughts and feelings OUT onto paper and finding clarity.*

You may be saying, "I don't know what to say. What do I write about?"

Well, I've found that it's best if you can be honest – what are you thinking and feeling right now?

You will find that the more you journal about your thoughts and emotions, the more you'll be able to RESPOND appropriately to those around you, rather than reacting badly out of your grief and pain.

At different times, I kept a journal of how I was feeling on particularly bad days, and I would just write and write and write. I would never reread it. It didn't matter what I wrote or if it even made sense. I just wrote out ALL of the frustration and anger and sadness (and every other emotion) onto paper. And in the end, I felt better, and my mind became clear.

SPEAK TO PEOPLE

Journaling works hand-in-hand with talking to people, particularly for those of us who prefer to have someone to talk to. **It's not one or the other; you need both.**

- **Speak to trusted friends**. Choose wisely. Not everyone is trustworthy, and many people won't know how to handle your negative emotions, others may not feel confident to deal with them. But a trusted friend who can empathize with your journey and encourage you to KEEP MOVING FORWARD is a gift.
- **Speaking to your kid**s can be tricky because we don't want to overburden them with our emotions. So, how much is too much? **My rule of thumb is to tell them enough to include them in your process, but not so much that you burden them.**
- **Make yourself available for kids to talk to you.** Let your children know that you're available for them to speak to you. Let them often know that you're here for them at any time for them to talk to you about their feelings and worries.

I remember telling the kids that I am here for them, that they can talk to me at any time, that I wanted to be there for them and help them with their worries.

KEEP YOUR THOUGHTS IN PERSPECTIVE

Thoughts, both negative and positive, come and go like fish in the sea. However, negative thoughts tend to confuse you about *who you are* and *what you're capable of doing*. You don't need additional confusion now.

For example, if you find yourself thinking, "I can't do _____," don't just believe it.

- Instead, write down all of the reasons you think why you CAN'T do that particular thing and then write down all of the reasons you CAN.
- Once you've finished your list: you may discover that the CAN'T-side is much longer than the CAN-side.
- Even if one of those CAN reason is *"because the children need me to do this,"* then that's a good enough reason to do it. If your kids need you to do something, then you will certainly find the strength to do it!

If you are struggling to work things out in your head, then write it down. Your brain can only do so much.

- Write down what challenges you are facing right now.
- Write down all of your options. What can you do? How can you do it?
- Work out what looks like the best solution at the moment, and put it into practice.
- If it doesn't work, it doesn't mean that you won't ever be able to do it. It may just mean that you need to change the plan slightly right now or try another option or you may recognize because of this process that you need to ask for help.

> *Try not to problem-solve when you're having a bad day. Negative emotions will only cause you to make decisions you may regret later. Rather wait until you're feeling a bit better.*

I remember keeping a list of things I needed to do. If I couldn't work things out in my head, I would at least work them through on paper. I realized that there were times that I just couldn't think or make decisions because of the fog of grief in my mind. On those days, I wouldn't even try. Instead, I acknowledged to myself that, "I feel unmotivated and that's okay." I knew it wouldn't last forever. A day or two later, I would pick myself up and try again.

And just as importantly, don't try to work everything out at once. Give yourself some time. Grief is not a sprint; it's a marathon. Little-by-little, step-by-step.

Grief is not a sprint; it's a marathon. Little-by-little, step-by-step.

CASE STUDY

Fiona was a 50-year-old widow. Her husband was ten years older, and they had a teenage son. Married for 20 years, Fiona adored her husband who provided for the family. One day her husband tragically died. Fiona through her whole married life was devoted to her husband and raising her son. She had to learn how to do everything now from paying the bills to budgeting and four months after his death she could not cope with her grief. Fiona experienced a range of emotions and cried often. She did not know if what she was experiencing was normal. Fiona felt guilty and declined invitations to catch up with friends as she thought people would think she should have moved on by now. When Fiona did cry and try to talk to friends they told her to start moving on. She found each day a struggle and her son became worried about her and took on the role of looking after her. During therapy, Fiona felt relief that her feelings were normal. Slowly she started to write about her thoughts and feelings in a private journal. Fiona also found that by starting a routine of basic self-care, coping with bad days was easier. And she realized that her son needed her to care for him and help him with his grief too. Over the following months, Fiona felt that as she also started to feel better. She found that she was adjusting to life without her husband. She no longer felt guilty for spending time with friends and discovered that while feeling sad she could also feel good within herself.

You can contact me on my Facebook Group – Dr Olga's Widows Guide to Grief https://www.facebook.com/groups/widowsguidetogrief

---

MY TIPS
Grief is a journey with no timeline. It's okay to grieve.
Try to eat well and do some light exercise.
If in doubt about your health, get a check-up.
Allow yourself the time to be mindful, observant of your emotions.
Pamper yourself to wash away tears.
Write in your journal to release your thoughts.

Self-care is important to help you manage your grief. It also allows you to show your children the importance of self-care.
So, take a deep breath and be kind to yourself today! You can do this.

IN MEMORIUM

The following photos are provided of my family in Memoriam of Mick. I provided these photos to put a face to the names so that our journey helps you to heal.

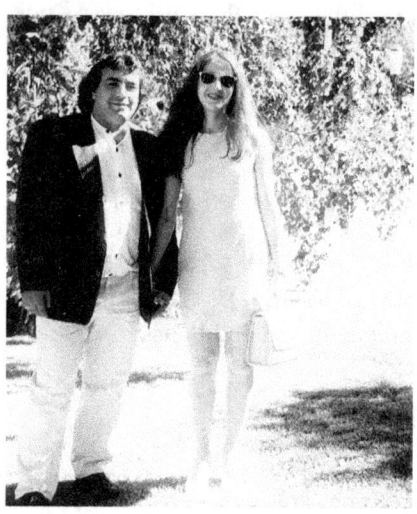

Mick and I at a wedding before we were married

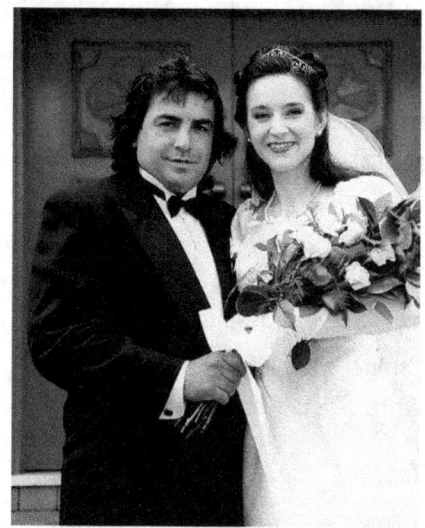

Our Wedding

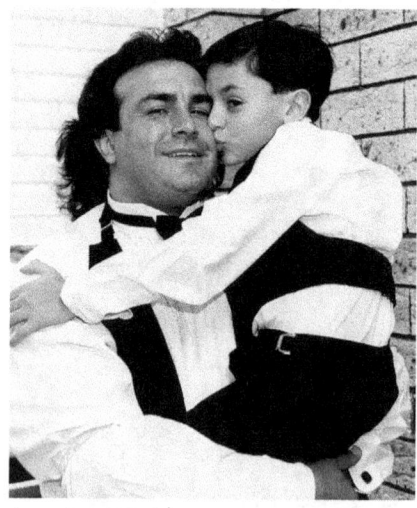

Jarred and Mick at our wedding

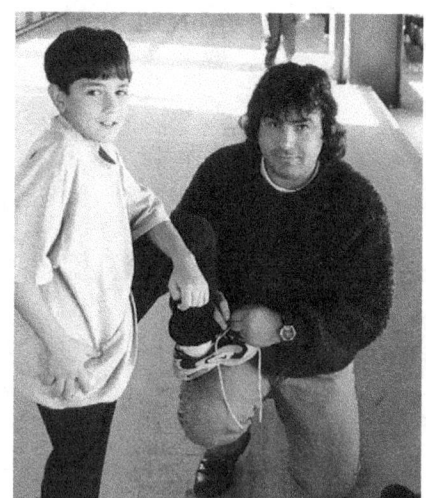

Jarred and Mick at an athletics carnival

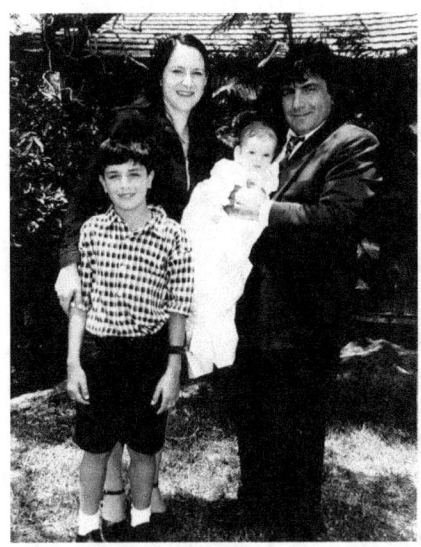
Alex`s Christening, Mick, Jarred and I

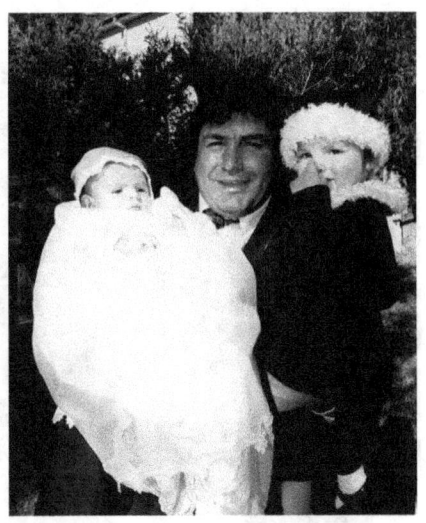
Mick holding Chloe and Alex at Chloe's Christening

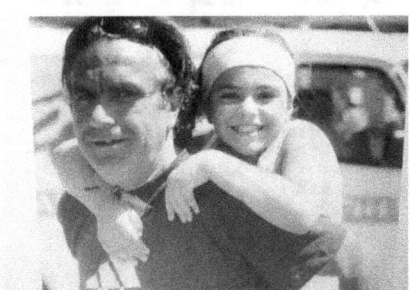
Mick carrying Chloe at the Athletics Carnival

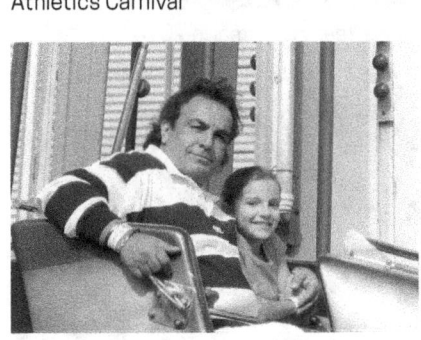
Mick and Alex on a ride at Sydney Luna Park

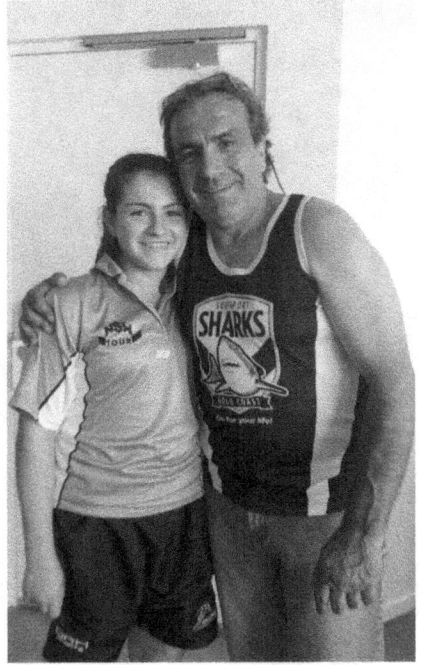
Mick with Chloe when Chloe was playing State basketball

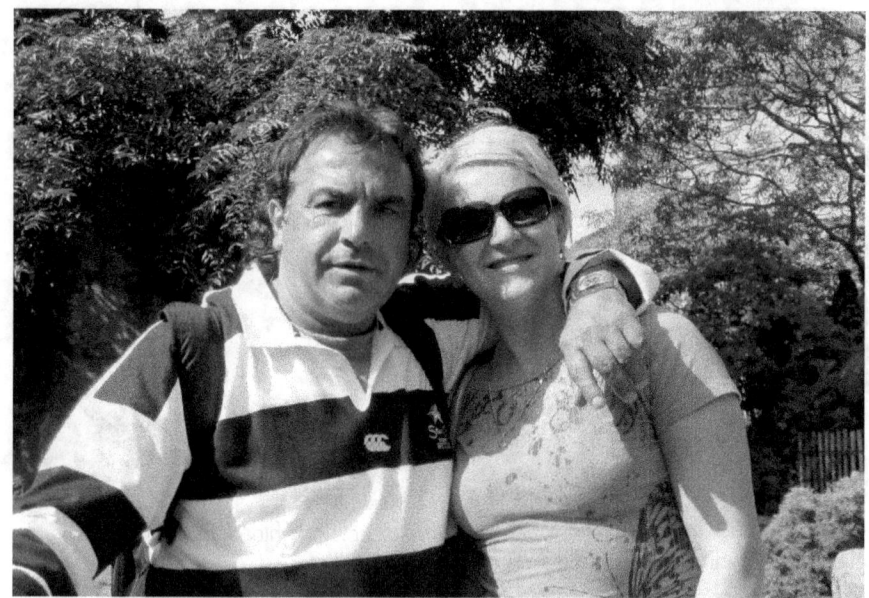

Mick and I

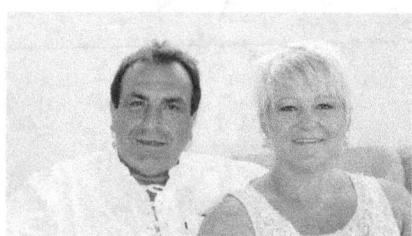

Mick and I 2014

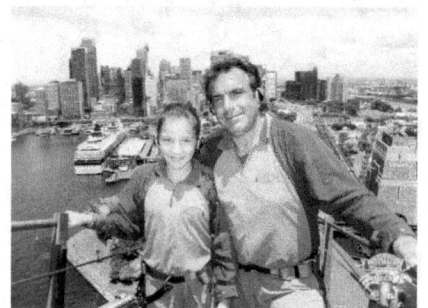

Mick and Alex Sydney Harbour Bridge Climb

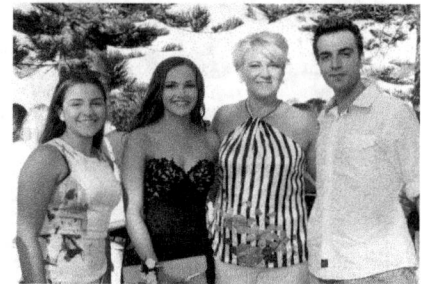

Alex's Year 10 Formal in 2014

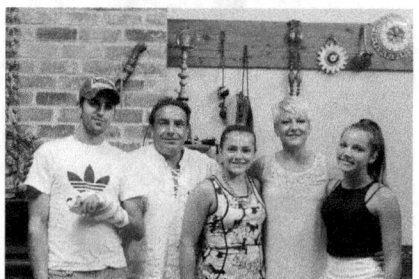

Family 2014

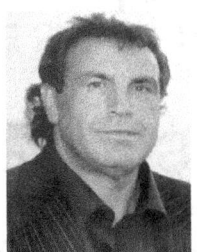
Mick

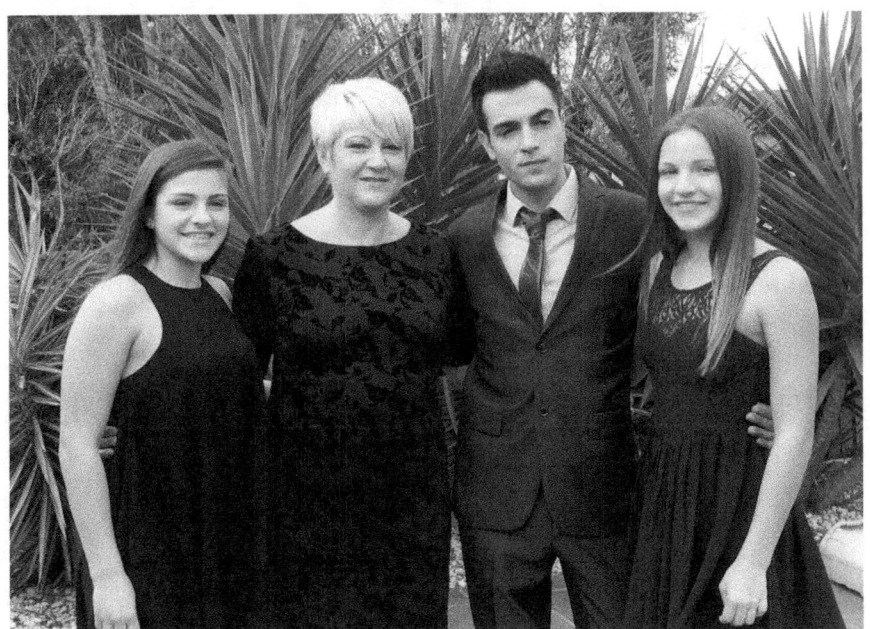
Mick's Funeral

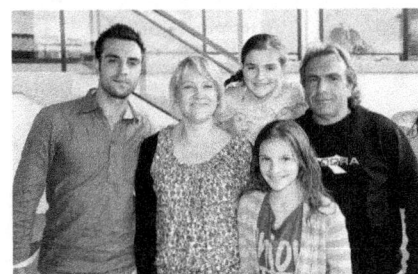
Family 2006

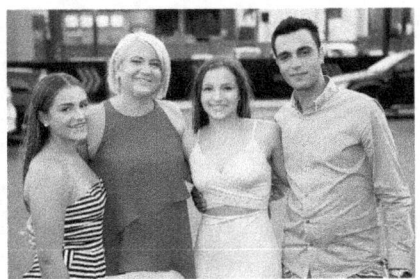
My surprise Birthday dinner 2016

CHAPTER 5

Those special days

"What we have once enjoyed deeply we can never lose.
All that we love deeply becomes a part of us."

~ Helen Keller

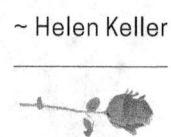

Milestones, one of the most inevitable and dreaded parts of our journey of grief. I remember the first milestone in my journey... Mother's Day. It had only been three weeks since Mick had passed away and I was in no mood to celebrate.

"What would you like to do for Mother's Day, Mum?"

"Nothing."

I knew it was coming, but I didn't care. My heart ached, and I just couldn't face a special day without him. I didn't want to go out for lunch or dinner, and I certainly didn't want to see others so happy, women with husbands, children with their fathers.

No, I wouldn't say that I was angry, nor jealous. I didn't hate other women who still had their husbands; that's just part of life. But my grief tore through me, and all I wanted was to be left alone with my tears. The pain was mine, it was my journey, and no one else could understand it or save me from it.

The only thing I wanted for Mother's Day was my children, and I already had that. I was so grateful that we'd had our children. They were such a blessing, and that was enough for me. In the end, apart from going to the cemetery to visit Mick, I spent Mother's Day no differently than the other 364 days of the year.

The only thing I wanted for Mother's Day was my children, and I already had that.

Milestones during grief are momentous for many reasons. Not only do they mark the passage of time, but they also slowly accustom you to your **New Normal**. Anniversaries, birthdays, holidays, festive seasons, and any other special days can trigger deep feelings of dread, sadness, and all the emotions that come with the harsh, piercing reminder of your loss.

I remember one of Mick's aunts saying to me, "*They never really leave you but walk beside you every day.*"

That phrase became such a comfort to me, despite the dread I would feel just before each milestone. I didn't even realize until much later how anxious and stressed I would get. I suppose I just wanted to include Mick in our special days and was desperate for all of our plans to work out 'perfectly.' Most often, our special days included visiting him at the cemetery and bringing him something special.

The reality is that, despite the incredible heartache you feel during this time, you have an opportunity to start to build new memories and create new traditions. It doesn't happen automatically, and it will take a year of 'firsts' to do this well. That means that for one full calendar year, you can re-invent special days and how you celebrate them as a family.

- What would your special days be like if you did the way you and your children wanted?
- How will you keep the memory of your loved one alive?

Despite the incredible heartache you feel during this time, you have an opportunity to start to build new memories and create new traditions.

These are some of the ways my family and I managed our milestones.

Father's day

Every Sunday morning, Mick would go to the local bakery to buy croissants and sultana pastry snails for our family breakfast. So, for Father's Day, we kept his tradition. We went to the cemetery to have breakfast with him, bringing a fresh bouquet of flowers, croissants and sultana pastry snails, a cappuccino for me, and a latte for him (that was his favourite). It was lovely! We sat on a blanket, enjoyed casual conversation, and celebrated our special Father's Day with him.

As we left the cemetery, I was amazed at how relaxed I felt. I understand that anxiety is normal, but I wondered to myself, *"Why was I so anxious? What's to be afraid of?"* I still don't have the answer maybe it was my fear of how I would cope.

Birthdays

Celebrating birthdays, both yours and theirs is another significant event. It's sad to mark the passage of time and not have your loved one with you.

For Mick's birthday, we chose to do what we usually did, and that was to go out for dinner. For our birthdays, we would do the same. We also wanted to remember him by being physically close to him in the way that we could and for us that was going to visit him at the cemetery.

Our family tradition is to have your loved one embalmed and placed in a crypt. Other's may have a plot in the cemetery or have created a special place for their loved one; for example, have planted a tree in memory of their loved one or have made a garden. Regardless of where your special place is, spending time there allows you to have some closeness with your loved one.

Christmas

I remember our first Christmas without Mick so clearly. Once again, I experienced waves of anxiety, sadness, and fear leading up to the day, fear about how the children would cope.

I kept our tradition alive of putting presents under the tree for them while they were asleep. It doesn't matter how old they get; they still like to get up in the morning and find presents under the tree. But this Christmas, they also got a special gift from their dad. He had wanted to surprise them with an iPhone that year, so in his absence, I followed through with his plan. The look on their faces and the smiles from ear-to-ear were the best gifts. I told them that I was honouring what their father promised them from the beginning of the year.

That year, our extended family went away for the holidays, and we were able to spend a quiet Christmas alone. First, we visited Mick at the cemetery and hung Christmas ornaments on the flower vases. Then we went down to the beach and enjoyed a quiet, relaxing day together. It was a very special time.

Wedding anniversary

On our 18th wedding anniversary, the sadness was overwhelming. I just wanted to be alone. I felt flat and unmotivated, and just couldn't 'do' anything. I cried on and off and then went down to the cemetery with a beautiful arrangement of flowers. Mick's favourite colour was blue, so I made sure to include blue flowers in the bouquet.

I sat for a long time at the cemetery with him, sometimes crying, sometimes talking to him, and sometimes just soaking in the silence. At one point, I remember telling him that I was going to "visit his new friends" (which is what I called the other deceased people at the cemetery). I walked around for a while looking at the other graves and reading their plaques. Some of the 'friends' were old when they died, some middle-aged, and some were children or babies.

And I wondered to myself, *"How did they die?"* and *"How did their loved ones cope with the pain of separation?"* Somehow, walking around the cemetery always gave me a sense of peace and helped me to feel calm again.

Easter

Mick died on the 19th of April, 2014, which happened to be Easter Saturday that year. In hindsight, I can see now how extraordinary that particular Easter was.

Traditionally at Easter, we have lunch with our family on Easter Sunday, but that year, Mick insisted that we invite his family on Good Friday instead. That was odd; we never did anything on Good Friday. I wasn't keen to change our plans because I was working late on Thursday and couldn't do the required shopping and preparing. However, when I came home from work that Thursday, not only had Mick done the grocery shopping, he had also done all the washing and had even mowed the lawn. (Now you've got to understand something about Mick he hated mowing the lawn. For him to mow the lawn without us nagging him, he must have badly wanted a Good Friday lunch.)

So, we had a lovely Good Friday lunch with the family and took lots of family photos. Afterwards, he kept to himself stating that he was feeling tired. I didn't think anything of it at the time.

Weeks later as I was reflecting on our 'odd' Easter weekend, I had to wonder, *"Did he know he was going to die? Is that why he changed Easter Sunday lunch to Good Friday?"* My personal feeling is that *"Yes, He knew,"* and that's why he did it. He was preparing me for the inevitable and wanted to make sure I would be okay and know what to do. I'm so grateful for that.

At one point, I remember the children saying that *"*Easter will never be the same." I gently corrected them, saying, "No, Easter will always be Easter. The nineteenth of April will not always fall on Easter weekend, and although it brought pain and sadness in 2014, it won't always be so." It was important to me that they not associate Easter with the pain of losing their father.

Today, we continue to celebrate Easter in our usual way. We go to the cemetery in the morning to visit Mick and wish him a "Happy Easter," and then we enjoy our Easter Sunday lunch with his family.

Twelve month anniversary

As the anniversary of Mick's death approached, I started experiencing those familiar feelings of anxiety again. On the outside, I thought I was okay, but subconsciously I was stressed, scared that I would forget him after twelve months, just like many of my clients had shared their fear of forgetting. Suddenly, I knew exactly how they felt. While I never feared I would forget what he looked like, as we have a photo of him in our family room, many of my clients feared just that, that is forgetting what their loved ones looked like or the sound of their voice.

I knew that, logically, my mind would never erase him; I could never forget him. But the fear of forgetting him tormented my mind. *"Will I have to remind myself constantly that I was married to him? Will I have to remind myself that Mick was my husband?"*

> *I knew that, logically, my mind would never erase him; I could never forget him. But the fear of forgetting him tormented my mind.*

NO, you never forget! What a relief to find that he regularly pops into my mind. I will always remember him.

It's our family custom to have a church service on the twelve-month anniversary in remembrance of your loved one. On this significant day, I invited family and close friends to attend a church service and then join me for lunch. This precious time together was the perfect conclusion to our first year of grief.

TIPS FOR DEALING WITH MILESTONES

As you prepare yourself for a year of 'firsts,' here are some helpful tips to keep you healthy and calm through the process.

Beforehand:
- Make a note of significant days that may be difficult for you.
- As they approach, start thinking about what you want to do, and how you will manage and look after yourself on that day.

On that day:
- Don't expect too much from yourself.
- Permit yourself to 'not be OK.'

Suggestions to make the day special:
- Create a memorial that has significance to you
- Write a letter to your loved one
- Visit a favourite landmark
- Visit family and friends

- Make a scrapbook, or create a personalized photo album
- Do something your loved one enjoyed
- Plant a tree

Remember, milestones often stir up many negative emotions. You are normal. That's why it's important to do something that makes you feel good. Something as simple as going for a walk, getting a massage, watching your favourite movie, reading a magazine, or just taking a long, relaxing bath.

Remember help is always available. Join me for support on my Facebook Group – Dr Olga's Widows Guide to Grief https://www.facebook.com/groups/widowsguidetogrief.

> *Remember, milestones often stir up many negative emotions. You are normal. That's why it's important to do something that makes you feel good.*

As you keep looking after yourself, especially after milestones have stirred up negative emotions, it's crucial that you're there for your children to support them during these times. It's also important to teach your kids to look after themselves as well.

CASE STUDY

Kellie was a 42-year-old widow with two boys 11 and 13 years old. After her husband's diagnosis with an incurable illness, he passed away two months later. Kellie had come to treatment as she felt she was not coping being a single parent and she became anxious and worried that she was not dealing with her husband's death and the effect this would have on her children. During her therapy, Kellie had become anxious as the anniversary of her husband's death approached. She saw the day as being sad and gloomy and was scared of forgetting her husband in the years to come. While Kellie's feelings were valid, she also found that as the upcoming anniversary neared, her anxiety increased. Kellie found that taking the time to plan the day with her two boys and creating something special that they all wanted to do had helped her and the kids to reduce the anxiety. Kellie found spending time with her sons had been nice, they reminisced about the past and Kellie, and her children have now decided that they will spend the day doing the same thing each year.

While we think about our 'firsts,' there are many firsts for our children. My daughter Chloe spent a lot of time with her father shopping. Mick also supported her at basketball.

I remember after Mick's death Chloe was playing with her representative team. She played well in the game, but I noticed that at one stage she had tears running down her face. While I couldn't talk to her during the match as the parents were always expected to be away from the girls, I asked her after the game if she been hurt as I'd seen the tears. She said she found it hard playing her first representative game without her father. She had been very anxious before the match and had found her emotions were overwhelming because she just wanted him to be proud.

Chloe reminded me that she'd told me she was anxious before the game. I felt instantly guilty that I'd misunderstood. "I thought you were worried about the match," I said, "I 'didn't realize."

Chloe's response was heart-wrenching, telling me how much she missed her father.

I sometimes wondered "Should I have done more, or read into it more?" I can only say that Chloe and I hugged and cried together over our loss. I apologize deeply; I wish I could have done more.

I remember one of the 'firsts' for Alex was her Year 10 Graduation Dinner.

Many tears were leading up to it with her saying "I won't find a dress I like" "I won't look good," "everybody's got a dress except me...there's nothing I like". Deep inside I knew it was more about the anxiety of not having her father there. I often said to her "don't worry; your father won't let you be without a dress, he'll want his little girl to look the best."

We found a dress, and while she was initially happy as the graduation date neared, Alex said she didn't think she liked it and didn't think she would look good.

In the days leading up to the event, I hugged her, I talked to her and did as much as I could to help her prepare for the graduation dinner without her father being there. We acknowledged it would be hard to watch her friends with their father's.

I said to Alex "he'll always be watching from the skies above with a proud smile on his face." And so off she went happily with her dress, hair, and makeup. She told me afterward, she knew deep down he was with her.

I remember one of Jarred's 'firsts' was returning to his carpentry work after an injury at work. His father always guided him and was always there for him to discuss any issues with work. After Mick died, Jarred felt alone, anxious and overwhelmed, but he knew he had learned enough from his father and he had the support of others in the building trade if he needed any help.

Jarred did not talk as much about his emotions and firsts but this can be normal for adult children. As they navigate their world every day, you can only be there for them. I let him know that I would always be there for him.

While we continue our grieving journey, adjusting to our New Normal, we need to support and help navigate our children too through their firsts. In understanding the importance of not only our 'firsts' but the unique 'firsts' of our children, I've asked my beautiful children to bring their perspective to this book too.

> *While we continue our grieving journey, adjusting to our New Normal, we need to support and help navigate our children too through their firsts.*

In the following chapter, you will meet Chloe, Alex, and Jarred. You will learn a little more about them and their personal experiences as children who lost their father.

I asked them individually if they were willing to write about their experience for this book. Unanimously all the kids said yes. The wanted to share what happened to them in the hope that what they went through might help someone reading this book too.

As they began to write about their experience, I prepared them for the fact that deeper layers of grief would arise as they processed and wrote their story. My children were proud to talk about their father and have their journey included in this book. They too are adjusting to their 'New Normal' in the hope that you find yours.

CHAPTER 6

When there are children involved

"I truly never learned what the words **I miss you** were until I reached for my Dad's hand and it wasn't there."

~ www.yourtribute.com

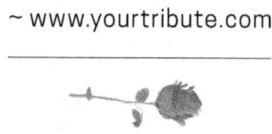

When I first learned of Mick's death, I remember asking myself, "*Oh my gosh! How do I tell the children? How do I soften the blow?*"

Unfortunately, there is no easy way to soften that blow you just have to tell them, grab them, pull them in tight, and hug them. That's what I did with each of them, following soon after with the words, "we'll be alright."

Even as I write this, I cannot imagine what their pain was like then and continues to be today. To be fatherless is heartbreaking, whether you are a teenage girl or an adult son. There are still so many special moments in the future that they would've loved to share with their Dad. Graduating from high school, university, going on their first date, getting their driver's license, getting married, having their first child. The list feels and seems quite neverending!

So, to understand their pain better myself, and to share this journey with you, each one tells their story. Our children's story has helped me to understand their pain at a greater level. As they share this journey with you I hope it will likewise help you on yours.

The following is what each of them said.

CHLOE WAS FOURTEEN YEARS OLD

The moment Mum told me Dad had died, I remember thinking, *"This is not real. What! My father's gone?"* and I started to cry. She grabbed me and pulled me tight. To me, it felt like he was only away on a weekend holiday and he'd walk through the front door at any moment.

But once reality sunk in, I was lost for words. I was a broken girl and had no words to describe my pain. I know Mum tried to ease the heartache in her way, but my pain was also for her, knowing that now she had to raise two girls on her own.

There were things I started to worry about that other kids didn't need to … like if something happened to Mum, we would have no one. I was also concerned about her well-being. How were we going to cope? How would we survive? But Mum assured us that everything would be okay and that she will always support us.

For many weeks I was lost for words. Saying goodbye to my Dad at the funeral was hard, and I felt sick knowing I wouldn't be able to see him again. Mum always said we were 'two peas in a pod,' inseparable. At the cemetery, as I released my dove into the sky, I sent my Dad a special message. *"I love you, Dad. You will always be my best friend. Please help Mum guide us."*

After the funeral and the wake, I had a sense of peace seeing how much everyone around my Dad loved him. We were all feeling the shock and pain of his death. I wasn't alone in my grief, and that was strangely comforting.

When I came home, reality hit me; everything at home reminded me of him. The house was cold, and I missed him terribly, but I also knew that Dad was in my heart, along with all the memories of the things we did together, and no one could take that away from me.

I also worried about significant days that were to come: birthdays, Christmas, Easter, Father's Day, and the anniversary of Dad's death. I was even afraid to go to my friend's homes because seeing them with their fathers made my heart ache even more. I no longer had a father who would take me grocery shopping, bike riding, or skateboarding. Even worse, I no longer had a father who would come to watch me play basketball. He had been my *'Number One Supporter.'*

I'm so grateful for the support of my family and friends as I coped with the loss of my Dad. My Mum, sister, and brother are my primary support network, and through their love, guidance, and encouragement, they have helped me survive this difficult time. As a result of their support,

I've been able to talk about my feelings,
I have a healthier lifestyle,
I live each day as if it's my last, and
I have a more positive outlook on life.

> *I love talking about Dad. I miss him so much, and I think about him every day. Everything I do now is not only for me but also for him, to make him proud (and I'm sure he is).*

Learning to live without him was a huge change in our lives. We had to take each day as it came, but we also used the pain to make us stronger people. We even moved houses eight months after the funeral, and each new day brings us a *new beginning* and a *new goal*. We know that he is still with us, and I can now see that we have a healthier outlook on life. As a family, we have grown closer together, adjusted, and know that Dad would be happy with his family.

ALEX WAS FIFTEEN YEARS OLD

When I found out Dad had died, it felt very surreal. *"My Dad?"* I remember asking my uncle. He told me what had happened, but I just couldn't believe that he was talking about *my Dad*.

Instantly, waves of emotion flooded me. How could this happen to my Dad who taught me so much, it can't be true? Why did he have to die so early? I still needed him!

I needed to tell him one more time how much I loved him. I was desperate to tell him how much I appreciated everything he did for me, and thank him for believing that I could achieve anything I wanted in life.

I so badly wanted to thank him for being the BEST father and for always being there for me; he gave me the world. I needed to tell him all this, but I couldn't. He was gone, and the pain was overwhelming.

After the funeral, my whole body felt numb. The funeral was a time to say goodbye, but I just couldn't. I was waiting to wake up from this horrible dream. It was hard to accept that we would never see Dad again and that's what made it worse for me. I wanted to remember the happy memories we had because there were lots of them. But instead, I kept thinking of the times I argued with him. I felt broken and guilty that I could not say sorry to him for all my mistakes.

The feelings of guilt went on for months and made it extremely difficult to cope. I felt lost. During a particularly difficult time, I remember saying to Mum, *"I wish I had died instead of Dad; it was all my fault he died."* I'll never forget the tears this brought to her eyes as she exclaimed, *"NO! I can cope with Dad's death, but I could never cope with yours."*

Mum patiently and faithfully helped me deal with my guilt. She told me what Dad believed about death, and then she would say, **"We don't have a choice when it's time for us to die."** My Nonna (grandmother) died seven months before Dad, and Mum said that *"He had to leave us to look after her because that was the type of caring person he was."*

As time has passed, I've coped better with my grief. I've come to terms with Dad's death and have accepted what has happened. I believe that *'Everything happens for a reason'* and although I don't know why he was taken away from us so soon, I find comfort in knowing that there was a reason.

I worried a lot when Dad died, but mainly about money. I was concerned about how Mum would financially keep up with our needs, especially since my sister and I were now completely dependent on her. I worried about how we would pay the utility bills on the house. I even worried about our future, how we would live, and how we would cope with such a loss.

My mother is the strongest woman I have ever known. Not only did she have to deal with losing her husband, my father, but she also had to support us and keep us moving forward in life. My friends were also very supportive and always there for me whenever I needed them. They helped me take my mind off things and always made sure I was okay. If it wasn't for my Mum, family, and friends, I don't know how I would've survived.

I know, deep down, that Dad had to go, but also that he's still watching and guiding us. I believe that 'Everything happens for a reason,' and I like to set goals and achieve them. I know that Dad would be proud of the choices I'm making in life today.

I know, deep down, that Dad had to go, but also that he's still watching and guiding us.

 I believe that 'Everything happens for a reason,' and I like to set goals and achieve them. I know that Dad would be proud of the choices I'm making in life today.

JARRED WAS TWENTY-FIVE YEARS OLD

I was at a friend's house when I received the call about what had happened to my Dad. I just couldn't believe my ears; that was the last thing I expected to hear. Straight away, I felt sick with shock and disbelief and kept thinking, *"This can't be true. He must have got it wrong."* After realizing the gravity of what I'd just heard on the phone, I felt confused and angry, and my heart ached. It felt as if someone cut it in half.

I started to worry about my future. Dad had guided me through work and life, and I felt completely lost knowing that not only had I just lost my father, I also lost my mentor, teacher, and best friend. I had a lot of plans for my future that I still wanted to share with him, but that was gone. I could always rely on him for help and support, and now that was gone too. I was heartbroken that he wouldn't be there for any future milestones in my life. I lost my mother when I was very young, and now my only parent was gone.

I was involved a lot with planning the funeral which made me happy; it gave me something constructive to do, and it felt good to help lay my Dad to rest. In the week leading up to the funeral, our home family and friends filled the home giving their condolences, so there wasn't much time to be alone.

While the funeral helped me to say goodbye, it hurt more knowing that he was indeed gone. Reality kicked in. After the funeral, people stopped coming over, and it was quiet; too quiet. I felt anxious and alone. I hated the pain of grief, and it wasn't long before I also became depressed and unmotivated, like I was living in a crazy world. At times, I was just in denial. *"This can't be happening."*

I started to think about my sisters and my Dad's wife, Olga (the woman I call Mum), and I wondered whether they would still include me as part of their family. I worried about what was going to happen. I spent a lot of time reminiscing about Dad and even wondering whether he was proud of me. I knew that he would want me to be even more of a role model to my sisters, and he would expect me to help more around the house, but I found myself torn between being there for my sisters, helping Mum, and feeling lost in this new life without my Dad.

I received a lot of support in that first year from family and friends. In the beginning, I would just try to keep busy to distract myself from reality, but it would always catch up during the quiet times. I ended up taking some time out for myself to reflect and rebuild my life which helped me to move forward.

I must admit, though, I disliked answering questions about what happened. That wasn't helpful at all. What helped me cope with my grief was getting back to a routine and focusing on the positive memories of Dad. I often talk to him in my mind, and I know he's always with me. I also have my Mum, Olga, and my sisters, and although I don't live with them, I see them every week for dinner. I know I'm not alone. As I read their stories, I just cried and cried. Yes, I knew about their worries, and I could feel their sadness, but I never really knew how they felt. I suppose, at that time, they were working out their feelings and the new world around them. I tried my best to create an environment where they could find expression, closure, and healing. At the end of the funeral, I even arranged for each of us (and their cousins) to release a dove as a symbol of life, hope, renewal, and peace. I also released a dove into the sky, and it was wonderfully cathartic.

What helped me cope with my grief was getting back to a routine and focusing on the positive memories of Dad.

I knew that I had to reassure Jarred that we were still family and he was still a part of this family. His father not being there doesn't mean the family unit breaks up; I was going to do my best to keep our family together. After the girls and I had moved, it took some time to find a regular evening to have dinner together, but we managed to make it work. Every Monday, I cook dinner and Jarred comes over. We told him straight away he was to make himself 'at home,' and I know deep in my heart that Mick would be happy that we are still one family unit.

> *I knew that I had to reassure Jarred that we were still family and he was still a part of this family. His father not being there doesn't mean the family unit breaks up;*

HELPING TEENS GRIEVE

I realize that you may be deep in the furrows of your grief and that there are some days when you can barely get out of bed. I understand. At the same time, remember that your children are grieving too. They need you even more now.

Be aware that all teens grieve differently.

Here is a list of common reactions that can be a part of a teen's grieving process when teens grieve. Remember grief is individual therefore your teenage child/children may not experience all these responses.

Common reactions to grief in teens
- They may experience shock and disbelief that the person has died.
- They may experience prolonged sadness that a parent is gone.
- They may experience increased memory loss or difficulty concentrating.
- They may express reluctance to go to school.
- They may get into frequent fights with others and exhibit disruptive behaviour.

- They may be difficult to get along with and uncooperative.
- They may exhibit hyperactivity.
- They may have an increased need for personal attention and may use positive or negative behaviour to get it.
- They may experience feelings of abandonment, insecurity, and safety concerns.
- They may experience increased feelings of fear, guilt, relief, anger, rage, regret, or confusion. They may experience heightened insecurity or social awareness, such as being concerned with appearing 'different' to their peers.
- They may question what is important and demonstrate a change in values.
- They may exhibit an increased preoccupation with death, often asking sensitive questions and want more details than you are comfortable giving.
- They may take on adult responsibilities, such as an urgency to check in on surviving parents, siblings, extended family, friends, etc.
- They may exhibit changes in relationships and family roles.
- They may experience increased need to be physically close to safe adults.
- They may experience physical changes, such as difficulty sleeping or changes in appetite (increased or decreased).
- They may also experience physical issues, such as headaches, tiredness, muscle aches, and nausea.
- They may demonstrate increased anxiety about the future.

[Australian Centre for Grief and Bereavement, www.grief.org.au .]

If at any time you require further help, you can ask questions and feel supported at my Facebook Group – Dr Olga's Widows Guide to Grief https://www.facebook.com/groups/widowsguidetogrief

I knew it was important to normalize the children's feelings. I never hid my pain from them, and I remember telling them when I felt unmotivated. I wanted them to realize that it was normal to feel the different symptoms of grief. So, I would ask them if they felt something like that too (or depressed, or angry, etc.)? If they saw me cry, I'd tell them that I was sad and missing their father. I'd explain that it was okay to cry and that I'd feel better afterward.

I knew it was important to normalize the children's feelings. I never hid my pain from them, and I remember telling them when I felt unmotivated. I wanted them to realize that it was normal to feel the different symptoms of grief.

Be there to listen and talk to them

It is important while you are grieving that you let the children know that you are still there for them with open arms. Teenagers want to know the truth; therefore, telling them the truth shows them that you are open and honest, and it allows you to keep open channels of discussion for them to ask questions. If teens don't want to talk, give them their space and respect their decision. However, make sure you regularly check to see that they are okay. Let them know that you are there for them at any time in case they do want to talk.

"I'm here for you, anytime" was my mantra. My children knew they could talk to me whenever they needed me, or even message me by phone if I was not at home. I regularly asked them how they were doing, and reminded them that "I'm here for you."

As parents, we all fear the dangers of our children getting involved with the wrong crowd and potentially with drugs and alcohol. This fear is even more pronounced when you know that they are suffering incredible pain because of losing a parent. I was so scared that one or more of them would start using drugs or alcohol to numb their emotions. Thankfully, they didn't.

Provide a normal routine

During periods of intense grief, young people need to feel safe and secure. One of the best ways to provide that security is to help them get back into their normal routine and encourage them to participate in their usual activities. What sports and hobbies did they enjoy before?

During periods of intense grief, young people need to feel safe and secure.

Teenagers also like to spend time with friends, and being involved in regular activities is an excellent opportunity to reach out for support.

I remember getting my children back to their usual activities as soon as they felt they were ready. I knew they had solid support systems on their teams and in their friendship circles, and it was a great place to receive help from others. I allowed them to spend as much time as possible with friends as I knew it was right for them.

Encourage children to create memories

Allowing teenagers to plan their beautiful memories will help with their grief. There are many ways they can do this, such as writing in a journal, making a scrapbook of their favourite photos, starting a blog, or designing a memorial. If they are artistic at all, they can even do some personal artwork that will express their feelings with more creativity.

One of the things I did for my kids was to take all our old family videos and transfer them to a DVD, then they could watch them whenever and wherever. There were videos of special times they had with their Dad, and videos of significant moments in their childhood. What a gift. These DVD's allow them to look back whenever they want to and remember their father.

Provide additional support leading up to special occasions and anniversaries

As we discussed in Chapter 5, it's important to help your children prepare for special events on the calendar: birthdays, holidays, and anniversaries, etc. I remember getting caught up in my world of preparing myself for those days, and there were times when I could barely handle my own emotions, never mind add theirs to the mix.

But ignoring the impending event won't stop them from worrying about it or feeling sad. Denial isn't a remedy. You will have to bring it up sooner or later.

So, what could you do?

- Face it head-on and let your children know that it's okay to feel anxious or apprehensive when special events are coming up. Their feelings are normal.
- Develop a plan for what you will do (see Chapter 5). Be precise and creative.
- Remain as pleasant as possible on that day, and focus on making new memories together that are just as enjoyable as the old ones.

On that day, I always planned for our celebration to be as beautiful as possible, and for us to remember happy times with their father. I also made sure we talked about normal things as if Dad was a part of the conversation.

Taking time to plan these new memories is one way to instill hope for the future as children adjust to their new way of living. Show them, little by little, that life will carry on, and they won't be sad forever.

HELPING 6 TO 12-YEAR-OLDS GRIEVE

Although young children may not understand everything about death and dying, they are certainly able to comprehend the basic concepts of grief. However, because of their emotional immaturity, it is common for them to experience increased fear about their death or a higher sense of responsibility for the death of their parent.

> *Although young children may not understand everything about death and dying, they are certainly able to comprehend the basic concepts of grief.*

Here are some common responses to grief in children between the ages of six to twelve years old.

Common reactions to grief in children (ages 6–12 years old)
- They may experience difficulty adjusting to their new life without their loved one. Many children even believe death to be reversible, or that it will only happen to other people.
- They may be very curious about all aspects of death and burial, often asking uncomfortably detailed questions to those around them.

- They may experience increased fear, often imagining death as a 'bogeyman' or 'ghost.'
- They may experiment with role play games in which they pretend to die.
- They may experience increased anger over the death, especially toward anyone who was involved (e.g., doctors, parents, etc.).
- In some instances, children may not exhibit symptoms at all. They may only absorb the reality of what has happened over time.
- They may be quick to blame themselves for the death.
- They may experience physical reactions such as difficulty sleeping, loss of appetite, decreased academic performance, headaches, etc.
- They may worry about grown-up issues, such as who will look after them if another parent or caregiver dies.
- They may take on adult responsibilities, such as 'parenting' younger siblings.
- They may 'act out' their feelings rather than talk about them.
- They may experience heightened insecurity or social awareness. For example, children may worry about appearing 'different' to their peers.
- Because they don't know many other kids who have lost a parent, they may also experience extreme feelings of isolation and loneliness.

[For more information, please see the Australian Centre for Grief and Bereavement, www.grief.org.au .]

Some tips for helping young children grieve

It's quite natural to want to isolate yourself at this time, but try to help your children stay connected with you and their deceased parent. Talk to them about their fears and worries, and make sure they have enough information to understand what has happened. Reassure them that they are not to blame, acknowledge their feelings, respect their way of coping, include them with any funeral preparations, and encourage them to create memories.

Having a parent die can significantly affect a child's view of the world and their sense of safety. It's not uncommon for children to worry about getting sick and dying themselves. If your child is demonstrating similar fears, it may be helpful to visit your family doctor for a check-up. Call the doctor in advance to explain the situation so they can prepare for any questions your child may ask.

While some children are very social and can express themselves verbally, others keep to themselves and struggle to communicate. Either way, allowing them to talk freely about what happened and what they experienced will greatly help with their healing.

You can encourage your children to express their grief by:
- Talking with them about their deceased parent,
- Making a memory box in which to keep the items that remind them of their mother or father,
- Give each child copies of select photos with their parent
- Making a scrapbook of memories,
- Allowing them to have a particular item that belonged to their parent (e.g., a piece of clothing, jewelry, or some other keepsake), and
- Creating new rituals as part of remembrance activities

It's important to meet your children's physical and emotional needs so they can feel cared for and safe. The best way to do this is to give them plenty of hugs. Ask family members and friends to also help with this. Have you ever heard the age-old adage, "It takes a village to raise a child"? Well, that is especially true when a child loses a parent.

Similarly, ask for extra support from their teachers at school. Explain the situation as soon as possible, and discuss options for getting your children the support they need. And try your best to get them back into their routine to help them develop a sense of safety and security.

With love and support from you, family, and friends, your children will be able to work through their grief. However, if at any time you are concerned about their well-being, do not hesitate to seek further help for them.

[NOTE: The same goes for you, too. If you don't take care of yourself physically and emotionally, you won't be able to take care of your child/children either. If you're struggling to cope with your grief, help is available. You can ask questions and feel supported at my Facebook Group –

Dr Olga's Widows Guide to Grief https://www.facebook.com/groups/widowsguidetogrief.

I add here a further piece of advice concerning how to help your children grieve?

 Grief takes time, and it is a process. Help your kids journey WITH you on your path to healing. Don't suffer in silence, and don't allow them to suffer in silence either. Use this precious time to grow closer and find comfort and healing together.

"Use this precious time to grow closer and find comfort and healing together."

Dr Olga

CHAPTER 7

Myths and what the widow does not want to hear

"And no matter what anyone says about grief and about 'time healing all wounds,' the truth is, this kind of sorrow never fades until the last breath, and the heart stops beating."

~ Tiffanie DeBartolo

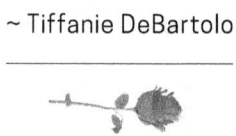

In the previous chapters, I have aimed to support and encourage you in your journey of grief. We've discussed what to expect, and how to handle all the different aspects of your life right now as you adjust to your NEW NORMAL.

As a Clinical Psychologist and a widow, I know there are many myths about grief. But there are also many things people say to widow's that we don't want to hear.

It is so important to keep reminding ourselves that grief is a journey, with no right or wrong way to grieve.

COMMON MYTHS

There are some common myths that many people believe about grief that sometimes keep us stuck expecting our journey to be the same. Perhaps these are beliefs that you grew up with, or maybe you learned them from teachers or peers. Regardless of where they originated, let's look at the myths and discover the truth instead.

Myth #1: grief and mourning are the same.
No, grief and mourning are not the same. Grief refers to the internal thoughts and feelings during a time of loss. It's those waves of emotion that overwhelm you without warning. Some sources define it as "keen mental suffering or distress over affliction or loss." (Dictionary.com)

Grief is the result of loving. If you didn't love your loved one and have a deep attachment to your loved one (or anyone and anything else you have grieved in the past), you wouldn't feel such pain.

Mourning, on the other hand, is the *outward expression of sorrow* for a person's loss. There are many ways different cultures expect widows to participate in bereavement. While these behaviours can change over time a common mourning symbol of expression for sorrow is wearing black.

Myth #2: grief follows a logical pattern.
No, there is no right or wrong way to grieve, and there is no set time frame in which to complete it. Each person's grief is uniquely their own, and it's certainly not predictable. Grief is the healing process that helps us deal with the loss of our loved one. Grief will ebb and flow throughout our lifetime, and while we don't ever 'get over' the loss of someone close to us, we do learn to live with that loss.

Myth #3: when I move on with life, it means I have forgotten my loved one.
This myth is simply rubbish. It's impossible to forget someone to which you were emotionally and spiritually connected.

Moving on means that you have accepted the reality of your loved one's death. You understand that they are not coming back, and that life must carry on. You are choosing to honour and respect their memory by creating a new life for yourself and your children and living it to the best of your ability. That is not the same thing as forgetting.

> *Moving on means that you have accepted the reality of your loved one's death. You understand that they are not coming back, and that life must carry on.*

Myth #4: the goal is to 'get over' grief.

As a Clinical Psychologist, I can attest to the damage caused by this myth. When people rush through the process of grief, they not only discourage themselves but they also inadvertently delay their healing. That delay then causes them to believe that there must be something wrong with them because it's taking so long to feel better.

Grief is a natural process, and you must allow yourself to feel the pain. Your thoughts and feelings are normal. **The aim is to go through the process of grief, patiently and thoroughly, and move into a new reality.**

Myth #5: friends and family can help by not bringing up the subject of grief and loss or our loved one.

Some people feel very uncomfortable with grief. They don't want to make you feel sadder than you already are, so they avoid the subject altogether. Another thing people can sometimes do is attempt to make you feel better by overly praising you. They might say "You're so strong," or "Keep busy."

While their hearts are usually good and kind, this only results in the widow grieving alone. They start to feel that they can't express their emotions in front of other people, and they end up missing out on the support of family and friends.

Talking about your loss is important. Perhaps even give yourself permission to bring the topic or the name of your loved one up as it feels right for you. It will help you grieve and will assist others to know it's safe for grief to happen.

Myth #6: staying busy will keep the pain away.

Staying active won't protect you from suffering. All it does is delay the inevitable. You need to give yourself time, space, and permission to grieve properly. Allow yourself to feel, cry, get angry, laugh a little, and then shed more tears. If you don't allow yourself to grieve now, it will catch up with you sooner or later.

Myth #7: if I cry, I'm weak.

Not true. Crying is a natural response to pain.

Feeling sad or upset does NOT mean you are weak. In fact, it's much more harmful to deny pain and suppress emotion. Allowing yourself to cry relieves those pent-up emotions and facilitates the grieving process.

> *Allowing yourself to cry relieves those pent-up emotions and facilitates the grieving process.*

Myth #8: if I don't cry, it means i'm not sorry for my loss.

Yes, crying is a healthy response to the sadness, but it's not the only response. There are some people who, for one reason or another, never cry. But it doesn't mean they don't feel grief. They may just have other ways of dealing with it.

Who are we to judge whether or not someone is sorry for their loss? Be careful not to make judgments toward yourself or others. That's just unfair and unwise.

Myth #9: grief should last about a year.

Who says? There is no time frame for grief. For some, it may only take a couple of months; for others, it may take years. There is no rule when it comes to grief. Everyone's experience will be different.

Myth #10: 'moving on' means I forget my loved one.

No, No, No! You will never forget them. They will always be with you and in your thoughts. Moving on means you've accepted your loved one's death, and you are choosing to continue to live. They wouldn't want you to stop living, would they? When you make a new life for yourself, you keep the memory of your loved one alive.

What a widow does not want to hear

This chapter wouldn't be complete if we didn't also address some of the irritating and annoying things that people say to widows. **Often, it's just because they don't know what to say and feel. People often need to 'fill the space'.**

As a Clinical Psychologist in the years before and since my husband's death. I have asked clients who had experienced the loss of their loved ones to identify the things people had said to them that they didn't find appropriate. Or if there were specific things people told them that had evoked anger or triggered something unhelpful. I've included a summary here along with my personal experiences since my husband's death.

Personally, I remember people saying things that were potentially inappropriate; however, I understood what they'd meant to say. Other times I recall thinking to myself later: *"What a thing to say."*

Following is a list of things not to say to a widow and what you can say instead.

"You're strong."
Says who? Why does the widow have to be strong? It's almost like saying she isn't allowed to grieve, express her feelings, or cry. When you think about it, why would a widow be 'strong' given she's just lost her loved one?

Grief is normal. If you don't grieve now, you will grieve later, and it could be at a time later when you're least expecting it. Now is the time the widow needs to rely on others for help and strength.

Instead say, "I am saddened by your loss, I care about you, and I am here for you" or "I'm very sorry you are going through this."

"You have to stay strong for the children."
What does 'strong' even mean? It's like saying, "You're not allowed to grieve." When a widow allows her children to see her grieving, it helps them understand and normalize their feelings. It's not a bad thing. It will also give her an opportunity to talk to her children about how they are feeling about their loss and will facilitate healthy expression of sadness.

The widow is doing the best she can under the circumstances, and again, this is the time for her to rely on others to help her with the children. She doesn't have to carry the whole responsibility alone.

Instead, say "What would you like me to do for the children at this moment" or "Is there something I can do to help with the children at the moment?" Be specific; ask what they need even asking about the fundamentals for example 'Have you had anything to eat?'

"He was too young to die."
Really? I think we all know that. A statement like this only makes the widow feel worse. She already feels intense pain, and these words only make her look for more reasons why her loved one died so early.

Instead, say "I am so sorry for your loss." It's essential to keep it simple and validate their feelings.

"Call me if you need anything."
While these words are intended to mean a willingness to help, at the time, a widow has no idea what she needs. Even if she did, she probably wouldn't ask for help. It's best to ask a family member or her best friend for suggestions on how you can help.

In all honesty, the widow needs practical things: cooked meals (frozen), fruit and vegetable baskets, help with the laundry and ironing done, her house cleaned, and the lawns and garden tidied.

Instead, say "Will you be home on Saturday? I would like to come and… (bring over some frozen meals)" or anything else you know is needed.

"Time will heal."
I'm about to let you in on a big secret… a widow never heals.

Yes, the pain will eventually soften, but she will live in a constant flux of emotion: sad, happy, sad, happy. Her loved one's death will always be a part of her.

Many widows have said that their only goal was just trying to survive that first year, the year of firsts (Please refer to Chapter 5). In the second year, she will further assess her loss because she didn't just lose a husband/partner, the widow is also now having to reassess emotional and financial security, the potential loss of some friends or family, and life as she knew it.

Instead, say «I wish I had the right words. Just know I care."

"He's in a better place."
This platitude is common; it slips off the tongues of many people who are trying to comfort their grieving friend. I understand that they want to convey compassion and concern, but, these words don't help. The only 'place' a widow can fathom at the moment is exactly where she is right now. She doesn't want him to be in a better place; she wants him to be home with her. Her great loss has led to enormous pain and strong feelings of loneliness and isolation in the big world around her.

Instead, talk about the widow's loved one, share your memories, or share a significant value he had, for example, caring so much for his family. Communication like this will help keep his memory alive.

"Did he have a will?"
Are you kidding me? This question is shocking. Let me be very clear here – unless they are a family member or a very close friend; this is NONE of their business! You do not have to answer this question.

Do not even ask this or raise this. It is simply not something a widow thinks you need to know.

"What are you going to do now?"
Who knows? Please don't ask this question. The widow only wants to take a nap and wake up to find that this wasn't real, that she has awakened from a nightmare. She is still trying to work out how she will manage to live through another day. Making decisions about the future will come eventually, but only once the initial shock and trauma have passed.

Instead, say "Is there anything you want to talk about?" or "I'm listening.…"

"I know how you feel."
Uh, excuse me? No, you don't. No one does. Even if they had experienced similar circumstances, no-one could know how you feel right now. Not even another widow can truly grasp how you feel. No one will comprehend the depths of relationship you had with your loved one. Everyone grieves differently.

Instead, say "I can't imagine how you feel, my heart goes out to you?"

"Don't cry."
Why not? You've just lost your husband, your spouse, your lifelong partner. I'll let you in on another big secret… a widow will always cry. It may happen at different times, and it may lessen in intensity as time goes by, but she will surely cry. Most often, she will cry in the privacy of her own home, but no one can tell her not to cry.

Instead say "I wish there was something I could say or do to ease your pain"

WHAT TO SAY TO A WIDOW

I realise that many people are often unsure of what to say to a grieving widow. That's why the mood becomes awkward, and conversation stops when she enters a room.
- They don't want to upset her or cause her more pain.
- They are uncomfortable with the intensity of emotion around her.
- Or they simply don't know what to say.

What is helpful?

Sometimes, visiting the widow and just BEING THERE for her is one of the best things you can do. I understand that you want to say something to comfort her, but most times, just listening is enough.

Remember you can't take the pain away, but you can provide comfort and validate her feelings. Especially on special days and anniversaries.

Ask her what she WANTS and NEEDS. If she can't think of anything, offer suggestions. For example, ask if you can do 'laundry' or 'gardening,' and if she agrees, then keep your word and do it.

Remember to keep your visits short. Don't spend hours at the house, unless of course, she has asked you to stay. Even then, bear in mind that she also needs time alone to recover and recuperate.

Don't be offended if she doesn't want you to visit. Some widows desperately need privacy; others desperately want friends around them. Be sensitive to her needs. Everyone's experience is unique.

During those weeks of my most intense pain, I remember thinking how difficult it must have been for the people around me. What could they possibly say to lessen my pain? Deep down, I knew they were only doing their best, and it was difficult for them too. I could sense their concern by the tone of their voice when they genuinely asked me, "How are you? How are you coping?"

GENERAL COMFORTING WORDS TO SAY TO SOMEONE WHO IS GRIEVING THE LOSS OF A LOVED ONE

- "I'm so sorry."
- "I'm here for you anytime."
- "I don't know what to say." It's okay, tell the truth. The widow will appreciate that she can freely share because you are not trying to fix her or tell her what to do.
- "I'm sorry for your loss."
- "My condolences."
- "I'm listening."
- "I'm very sorry you are going through this."
- "You are in my thoughts and prayers."
- "I wish there was something I could say or do to ease your pain."
- "Before saying anything else, I want you to know how sorry I am to hear of your loss."
- "My heart goes out to you during this period of grief and readjustment."
- "Is there anything you want to talk about?"

ONE FINAL WORD OF ADVICE WHEN REACHING OUT TO A WIDOW

Remember, what you can say to a widow in her grief greatly depends on your relationship with her (how close you are). The closer you are, you can say more intimate things and ask more personal questions. Just be sensitive to how she is coping right now.

Don't be too distant, nor overly familiar. Be genuine and sincere.

CASE STUDY

Megan, a widow of two months, was finding it hard to cope with the loss of her partner of 15 years. She cried regularly and was not sleeping well. After her partner died, she was told by family and friends that 'she had to be strong.' Megan started to believe that if she cried when family and friends were around, she was not being 'strong' and coping. She felt she couldn't grieve in front of family and felt alone. Megan also started to think that she was not grieving in the right way. Megan also had two adolescent children, and her parents told her it's "no good to cry in front of the children, you 'have to be strong' for the kids." She then began to feel guilty for grieving in front of the children. Therapy progressed from understanding grief and it being an individual response, to understanding her beliefs about being strong and working through her guilt.

CHAPTER 8

Twelve months on. Now what?

"Sometimes you have to accept that certain things will never go back to how they used to be."

~ Author Unknown

So, fellow widows, we've reached this stage of our journey together. We've survived the immediate shock of our loss, and we've learned healthy ways to deal with our emotions. We've prepared for and attended our loved one's funeral, and we've successfully navigated a year of 'firsts.' And most importantly, we've learned to look after ourselves as well as be there for our children.

And now, twelve months have passed, and you are probably asking yourself, *"Now what?"*

I'm about to let you in on another big secret, one that I wish the rest of the world knew…

Grief never ends; you just learn to live with it.

No, your grief will never end completely. It will come and go, and of course, the intensity of your experiences will vary, but this is part of your story, and it always will be. Living as a single parent WITHOUT your loved one is part of what makes you 'YOU.'

This journey is your NEW Normal.

NEW NORMAL. WHAT DOES THAT EVEN MEAN?

In Chapter 7, I said that "A widow never heals." No, I wasn't trying to be cruel or negative. I was merely stating the obvious… it is impossible to go back to 'what was.' The reality that you experienced with your loved one changed forever, and what's left in its place is what I call your "New Normal."

> *The reality that you experienced with your loved one changed forever, and what's left in its place is what I call your "New Normal."*

Rather than wasting time trying to turn back the clock, this New Normal is your opportunity to re-invent yourself in all areas of life. It's time to learn and grow.

You are re-inventing yourself in areas such as,
- Your new ability to manage household affairs (bills, gardening, maintenance, etc.).
- Your new way of interacting with friends and family.
- Your new way of spending your free time (evenings, weekends, and holidays).
- Your new way of approaching the future.

Who do you want to be in five years' time? Ten years? These are questions that we all need to ask ourselves as the years pass. Life goes on, and we must keep adjusting to our New Normal.

YOU NEED TO BE YOUR CHEERLEADER

Re-inventing your New Normal and dreaming for the future is something that will continue for the rest of your life. There will be many more adjustments to come and many more significant events. For example, when the kids finish university, when they get married, when they have their first child or any other milestones in their lives. (Not to mention, other milestones in YOUR life. Is there something you'd like to accomplish? Is there something you'd like to learn or do?)

While these happy events in your life may also bring brief moments of sadness, it's crucial that you praise yourself for what you are doing well.

- Look back and remember how far you've come.
- Look at how you've grown and dealt with your grief.
- Look at how you've handled problems and challenges.

Be proud of how far you've come, and the strength and courage you have developed within yourself along the way. Most importantly, be proud that you found the determination and fortitude within yourself to deal with your grief, no matter how hard it was or how impossible it seemed.

"Grief is not a sprint; it's a marathon. Little-by-little, step-by-step."

You HAVE done this.
You CAN do this.
And you will CONTINUE to do this.

With time, as you may have noticed by now, your steps and pace will quicken, and the path you're walking will become easier.

But what happens when some paths are harder to walk than others? What happens when grief continues to be overwhelming and unmanageable?

PERSISTENT COMPLEX BEREAVEMENT DISORDER

Sadly, some people experience unusually disabling or prolonged responses to the loss of their loved one. This reaction is a serious condition, referred to as Persistent Complex Bereavement Disorder.

In his article entitled "Persistent Complex Bereavement Disorder DSM-5," Dr. Kevin Fleming described the disorder in this manner:

"Formerly known as complicated grief disorder, persistent complex bereavement disorder causes sufferers to feel an extreme yearning for a deceased loved one, usually over a prolonged period. Feelings of longing accompanied by destructive thoughts and behaviours, as well as general impairment in resuming a normal life."

For such people, intense emotions cause extreme distress and impair them from coping with daily activities. Their grief responses become unusually long with little to no improvement.

Symptoms of persistent complex bereavement disorder

According to the *DSM-5 Grief Scorecard*, by Dr. J.C. Wakefield, someone suffering from this may or may not display the following symptoms:

- Indefinitely yearning/longing for the deceased.
- A preoccupation with focusing on the circumstances of the deceased's death.
- Intense sorrow and distress that does not improve over time.
- Difficulty trusting others.
- Depression.
- Detachment and isolation.
- Difficulty pursuing interests or activities.
- A desire to join the deceased.
- Persistently feeling lonely or empty
- Impaired ability in social, occupational or other areas of life.

While the above symptoms are also characteristic of normal grief, those suffering from Persistent Complex Bereavement Disorder will experience these symptoms for at least six months or longer.

If you recognize some of these symptoms, please do not diagnose yourself. Seek professional help immediately for a proper diagnosis and personalized care.

ADVICE FROM MY FATHER

I grew up with a father who was always telling me,

> *"Olga, you have to study so that you can get a good job. You need to know about money and your financial situation. You need to be independent and be able to look after yourself. Don't just rely on a man to take care of you, because you never know what can happen in life."*

Little did I know at the time how much I would need that advice. I don't think my father had any idea how appropriate his advice would be to my life. I can still hear his words ringing in my mind, *"Olga, you need to be independent and be able to look after yourself."*

As a woman, I have been showing and encouraging my girls for years how to be independent and self-sufficient. Now, it is ME who is giving them good advice.

Reflection

I must admit that my heart tears as we reach this final moment. I trust that this book has been more to you than just another self-help book on grief. Writing my story and sharing it with you has been another chapter of healing in my life my private journey toward wholeness.

> *Writing my story and sharing it with you has been another chapter of healing in my life my private journey toward wholeness.*

What a privilege it's been to take this journey with each of you.

Here's what I have learned about grief.

I can personally confirm that there is no absolute order or certainty to the stages of grief. (Do you remember the theories I mentioned in Chapter 1?) I experienced many of the stages, but not necessarily all of them, and they certainly didn't come in any particular order.

Rather than forcing myself into any one theory, I accepted the reality of the loss and allowed myself to process the pain of grief in my timing.

I've also learned a lot about myself.

I found out that I could face adversity and deal with it. Without realizing it, I even used emotion-coping and problem-focused strategies.

I learned a lot from Mick as well. He had often said, "Life goes on, and you have to keep going because the world won't stop." It was also he who said, "Don't listen to what others say because it has nothing to do with them anyway." As a result, I learned that I am no longer attached to what people think, and I can recognize that my choices have been good.

"Life goes on, and you have to keep going because the world won't stop."

> *"Don't listen to what others say because it has nothing to do with them anyway."*

I've also learned that, while it's scary to get out of my comfort zone, I CAN DO THIS!

I can set goals for myself while remaining flexible. I don't always need a deadline to get things done. And when my decisions don't work out like I expected them to, it doesn't mean that I've failed. No, it just means that I need to change my action plan.

I've also learned the importance of 'Me' time.

I've learned that pleasing others wears me down. In fact, it's impossible to please everyone all the time, and they aren't going to please me all of the time either. That's ok; we all need to do what suits us. Sometimes, I just need to do what I WANT to do (and what I NEED to do) so that I can stay healthy.

Over time, I have adjusted to a world without my husband (and I keep on adjusting). It's been challenging at times, but through the process of embarking on this new life, I've found an enduring connection with him. I am not helpless; I am not alone. I discovered my New Normal.

One final thought

If there is one thing I remember from Mick, from the beginning of our relationship to the very end, he has always said to me, "You are my rock, the best thing that ever happened to me, I love you so much." Those words still put a smile on my face!

Whether you've had similar experiences or not, I want to leave you with these final thoughts from me:

One day you will look someone in the eye like I've learned to and say "I've lived through this and continue to do so, and it has made me stronger and more resilient." But even more so I know I am walking confidently in my journey ahead knowing I have done the best I can and hold no regrets. I cherish each moment and take in the beauty of things around me.

I thrive in my New Normal.

One day you'll find yours too.

An ode to a widow

Don't feel sorry for me because I know what it feels like to be at my lowest and slowly rise again

Don't feel sorry for me because this is life and I accept it

Don't think my grief has ended because I have decided to enjoy every moment of my life

Don't judge me because you just can't understand

Don't judge me because you don't know what is right for me

Don't tell me what to do because you're not walking in my shoes

Don't think it's ever over because grief comes back

Don't look at the past as a bad dream, it was real and will always be real

Don't listen to others when they tell you to get over it

Don't think for one moment that moving forward is forgetting him

Don't believe for one moment that I don't think about him every day

Remember to keep reaching for happiness – it's out there

Dr. Olga xx

Bibliography

Australian Centre for Grief and Bereavement. Available at: http://www.grief.org.au/ [Accessed 13 Dec. 2017].

Hall, C. (2011). Australian Psychological Society : Beyond Kübler-Ross: Recent developments in our understanding of grief and bereavement. [online] Psychology.org.au. Available at: https://www.psychology.org.au/publications/inpsych/2011/december/hall/ [Accessed 13 Dec. 2017].

Kübler-Ross, E. and Byock, I. (1969). *On death & dying*. New York, N.Y: Macmillan.

Shear, M. K., Simon, N., Wall, M., Zisook, S., Neimeyer, R., Duan, N., Reynolds, C., et al. (2011). Complicated grief and related bereavement issues for DSM-5. *Depression and anxiety*, 28(2), pp.103–17.

Stroebe, M.S., & Schut, H. (1999). The Dual Process Model of Coping with Bereavement: Rationale
and Description. *Death Studies*, 23(3), pp.197–224.

Theravive.com. (2017). Persistent Complex Bereavement Disorder DSM-5 – Therapedia. [online]
Available at: https://www.theravive.com/therapedia/persistent-complex-bereavement-disorder-dsm--5 [Accessed 13 Dec. 2017].

Wakefield, J. C. (2013). DSM-5 grief scorecard: Assessment and outcomes of proposals to pathologize
grief. *World Psychiatry*. Jun; 12(2): pp.171–173.

Worden, J. (2008). *Grief counseling and grief therapy*. New York, N.Y: Springer.

Endnotes:

1. Kübler-Ross, E. *On Death and Dying.* New York: Macmillan, 1969.
2. Hall, Christopher. "Beyond Kübler-Ross: Recent Developments in our Understanding of Grief and Bereavement." *InPsych*, December 2011. https://www.psychology.org.au/publications/inpsych/2011/december/hall/
3. Stroebe, M.S., & Schut, H. (1999). The Dual Process Model of Coping with Bereavement: Rationale and Description. Death Studies, 23(3), 197–224.
4. Worden, J.W. *Grief Counseling and Grief Therapy: A Handbook for the Mental Health Practitioner*, 4th Edition. New York: Springer, 2008.
5. Hall, Christopher. "Beyond Kübler-Ross: Recent Developments in our Understanding of Grief and Bereavement." *InPsych*, 2011.
6. Shear, M. K., Simon, N., Wall, M., Zisook, S., Neimeyer, R., Duan, N., Reynolds, C., et al. (2011). Complicated grief and related bereavement issues for DSM-5. Depression and anxiety, 28(2), 103–17.
7. https://www.theravive.com/therapedia/persistent-complex-bereavement-disorder-dsm--5
8. Wakefield, J. C. DSM-5 grief scorecard: Assessment and outcomes of proposals to pathologize grief World Psychiatry. 2013 Jun; 12(2): 171–173. Published online 2013 Jun 4. doi: 10.1002/wps.20053.

About the author

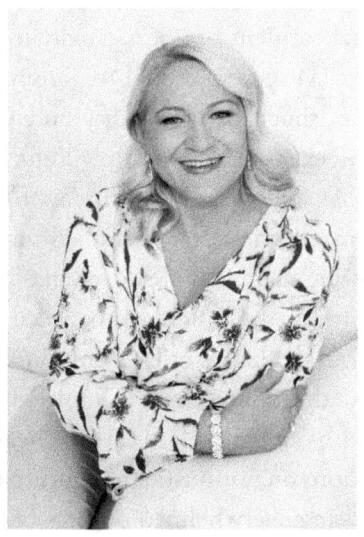

Dr Olga Lavalle is the Principal of Dr Olga Lavalle and Associates, a Psychology Practice near Sydney, Australia. Dr Olga understands grief from two perspectives, as a Professional and first hand as a widow after the sudden death of her husband in 2014. She weaves her Professional Psychologist's voice with the voice of herself as a mother and widow. Olga provides an honest and raw account of her family's journey through that first year as they adjusted to life without a husband and father. Whilst speaking of her journey, she provides practical strategies to help people through grief and real life accounts of how she has helped other widows.

As a Clinical Psychologist, Dr Olga Lavalle has over 30 years' experience working in Mental Health. Olga has worked in community mental health, inpatient mental health units, conducted research projects, and developed staff training programs. Olga has also co-authored many industry research papers and is regularly interviewed as an industry leader in the media.

Testimonial

Dealing with the mental torment of unexpectedly losing a loved one is an experience like no other. Mixed emotional responses flood our bodies and mind, ranging from ire, shock to incredulity and profound melancholy. Grief is inevitable; we all experience it at some point in our lives.

Dr Olga Lavalle's 'A Widow's Guide to Grief' is a must read, she addresses areas a person experiences when filled with overwhelming and intense emotions following the death of a loved one.

The guide also identifies the difference between suggested depression and grief; and although they share similar symptoms, they're not the same and should not be treated the same way; acknowledges the importance of remaining connected with our children to ease the healing process; as well as general tips and suggestions on optimistic thoughts to help us keep things in perspective and avoid being overwhelmed by fears of the future.

With a box of Kleenex, I've thoroughly enjoyed the guide and highly recommend it.

Dr. A. Gervaise MD

www.ingramcontent.com/pod-product-compliance
Lightning Source LLC
Chambersburg PA
CBHW050602300426
44112CB00013B/2035